THE LOST BOOK OF HERBAL REMEDIES

Discover Ancient Healing Secrets and Unlock the Power of Natural Remedies for Well-being

Nerissa Winslow

TABLE OF CONTENTS

CHAPTER 1: INTRODUCTION TO HERBALISM

Herbalism, an ancient practice rooted in the understanding and use of plants for medicinal purposes, has been a cornerstone of human health care across civilizations and cultures. This practice, often seen as the precursor to modern pharmacology, harnesses the natural compounds found in plants to treat, prevent, and manage a wide array of health conditions. The journey into the world of herbalism opens up a realm where nature meets health, offering a holistic approach to well-being that is both time-honored and increasingly validated by contemporary science.

Definition and History: What is herbalism? An overview of its history and significance across different cultures.

Herbalism is the art and science of using plants for therapeutic purposes. It encompasses the study of botany, chemistry, pharmacology, and traditional knowledge to understand how plant-based remedies can support health and wellness. Historically, herbalism has been a fundamental aspect of medical practices worldwide, from the ancient Egyptians, who documented their use of garlic, mint, and other herbs for healing, to the Chinese and Ayurvedic systems, which have developed sophisticated herbal pharmacopeias over thousands of years.

The significance of herbalism stretches beyond its medicinal applications, intertwining with cultural rituals, spiritual practices, and the daily lives of people. For instance, Native American tribes have used sage for purification ceremonies, while in Europe, herbs like lavender were used not only for their antiseptic properties but also to ward off evil spirits. This rich history highlights the diverse ways in which humanity has interacted with the plant kingdom, revealing a deep reservoir of knowledge and respect for nature's healing potential.

Basic Principles: Key principles of herbalism and how it differs from modern medicine.

At its core, herbalism is guided by principles that emphasize balance, holism, and the healing power of nature. Unlike modern medicine, which often focuses on treating specific symptoms or diseases, herbalism takes a more holistic approach, considering the physical, emotional, and spiritual well-being of the individual. This perspective is rooted in the belief that the body has an inherent ability to heal itself and that plants offer the necessary support to restore balance and health.

One of the foundational principles of herbalism is the synergy of plants. Herbalists believe that the complex mix of compounds in a whole plant or plant part can work together more effectively than isolated compounds. This concept, known as the entourage effect, suggests that the therapeutic impact of a plant cannot be fully replicated by a single extracted active ingredient. This holistic approach contrasts with the reductionist perspective of modern pharmacology, which often seeks to identify and use specific active ingredients.

Herbalism also places a strong emphasis on prevention and the maintenance of health, rather than just the treatment of disease. It advocates for a lifestyle that includes a balanced diet, regular physical activity, and the use of herbs as supplements to support overall well-being. This preventive aspect is complemented by the personalized approach herbalists take in recommending remedies, considering each person's unique constitution, environment, and health needs. As we delve deeper into the ancient art of herbal healing, we uncover not only the rich tapestry of traditions and practices that have shaped herbalism but also the modern resurgence of interest in natural remedies. This journey through the world of herbalism invites us to explore how ancient wisdom, combined with contemporary understanding, can guide us toward a more holistic and integrated approach to health and wellness.

What is herbalism? An overview of its history and significance across different cultures.

Herbalism, at its essence, is the practice of using plants for healing purposes. This tradition, deeply rooted in the fabric of human history, spans across millennia and continents, reflecting a universal human instinct to turn to nature for remedies to ailments and discomforts. The origins of herbalism are as old as human civilization itself, with archaeological evidence suggesting that even Neanderthals had knowledge of medicinal plants.

The historical journey of herbalism is a testament to the shared knowledge between generations and cultures. Ancient texts, such as the Egyptian Ebers Papyrus, dating back to 1550 BCE, detail over 850 plant-based remedies, illustrating the Egyptians' sophisticated use of herbs. Similarly, the Chinese Shennong Bencao Jing, written around 200-250 CE, lists hundreds of medicinal plants and their uses, laying the groundwork for Traditional Chinese Medicine (TCM). In the Western world, the works of Hippocrates and Dioscorides in ancient Greece laid foundational principles of herbal medicine that influenced European herbalism for centuries. Across different cultures, herbalism has not only been about the physical healing properties of plants but also their spiritual and psychological significance. For instance, Ayurveda, the traditional Indian system of medicine, integrates herbs into a holistic approach to health, emphasizing the balance between body, mind, and spirit. Native American healing practices, similarly, incorporate herbs in rituals and ceremonies, recognizing their power to heal not just the body but also the soul.

The significance of herbalism extends beyond its historical and cultural roots; it represents humanity's enduring relationship with the natural world. This connection, characterized by respect, knowledge, and stewardship, highlights the importance of plants in sustaining life and health. As societies evolved, so did the practice of herbalism, adapting to changes in medical theories, technology, and cultural beliefs. Despite these changes, the core essence of herbalism—its reliance on the natural world for healing—remains unchanged.

Today, the resurgence of interest in herbalism reflects a broader desire to reconnect with traditional ways of healing and a more natural lifestyle. This renewed interest is not a rejection of modern medicine but rather an acknowledgment of the complementary role that herbalism can play in achieving health and wellness. As we continue to explore the rich tapestry of herbal practices across cultures, we uncover valuable insights into how ancient wisdom can inform contemporary health practices, offering a more holistic and integrated approach to well-being.

Herbalism's history is a vivid illustration of humanity's quest for healing and well-being through the natural world. From the ancient Egyptians to modern herbal practitioners, the knowledge and use of medicinal plants have been a constant thread, weaving together the health and cultural fabric of societies around the globe. This enduring practice not only highlights the universal human reliance on nature's bounty but also underscores the importance of preserving this ancient wisdom for future generations.

Key principles of herbalism and how it differs from modern medicine.

Herbalism operates on a set of foundational principles that distinguish it significantly from the paradigms of modern medicine. At the heart of herbalism lies the belief in the healing power of nature, emphasizing that health and wellness can be achieved and maintained through the use of natural plants and herbs. This approach is holistic, considering the entire individual—body, mind, and spirit—in the quest for optimal health, rather than merely addressing isolated symptoms or diseases.

• Holism and Individualized Treatment: Herbalism views each person as a unique entity, with treatments tailored to the individual's specific needs, conditions, and constitution. This contrasts with the one-size-fits-all approach often seen in modern medicine, where diseases are typically treated with standardized protocols.

• Preventative Care: A key principle of herbalism is the emphasis on prevention. Herbalists advocate for a lifestyle that incorporates herbs not just for treating illness but as a means of maintaining health and preventing disease. This proactive approach to health is less emphasized in conventional medicine, which often focuses on reactive care.

• Synergy of Plants: Herbalism values the synergy of the whole plant, believing that all the components of a plant work together to provide a more balanced and effective remedy than isolated compounds. Modern pharmacology, in contrast, frequently seeks to identify, isolate, and synthesize specific active ingredients from plants for therapeutic use.

• The Healing Power of Nature: Herbalism is grounded in the principle that nature has an inherent ability to heal. Herbalists believe that by harnessing the natural properties of plants, they can support the body's own healing processes. This principle stands in contrast to the reliance on synthetic drugs and interventions characteristic of modern medicine.

• Education and Empowerment: Herbalism also places a strong emphasis on educating individuals about their health and how to maintain it using natural remedies. This empowerment enables individuals to take an active role in their health and wellness journey, differing from the more passive role patients often experience in the conventional healthcare system.

• Integration with the Environment: A deep respect for and understanding of the interconnectedness between humans and the natural environment is another cornerstone of herbalism. Sustainable harvesting practices and the ethical sourcing of herbs reflect this principle, highlighting a commitment to the health of the planet as well as the individual. Modern medicine, with its complex supply chains and reliance on synthetic chemicals, often lacks this environmental perspective.

CHAPTER 2: HISTORICAL OVERVIEW OF HERBAL REMEDIES

The tapestry of human history is rich with the use of herbal remedies, a testament to our enduring relationship with the natural world. From the banks of the Nile to the ancient cities of China and India, civilizations have long turned to the plant kingdom for healing and wellness. This chapter delves into the historical journey of herbal remedies across various cultures, tracing their evolution from ancient times through the Middle Ages and into the modern era.

Ancient Civilizations: Herbal Practices in Ancient Egypt, Greece, Rome, China, and India. The use of herbal remedies dates back thousands of years, with each civilization contributing its unique knowledge to the global compendium of herbal medicine.

- Ancient Egypt: The Egyptians were pioneers in the use of medicinal plants. The Ebers Papyrus, an ancient medical document, lists over 850 herbal prescriptions, including garlic for heart conditions and aloe vera for skin ailments. These remedies were not only physical but also spiritual, with herbs playing a crucial role in the embalming process and in rituals to honor the gods.

- Ancient Greece and Rome: In Greece, Hippocrates, the father of medicine, advocated for the healing powers of nature, emphasizing diet and herbal treatments. Dioscorides wrote "De Materia Medica," a comprehensive text that cataloged over 600 plants and their uses, influencing herbal practices for centuries to come. The Romans expanded on Greek herbal knowledge, incorporating it into their medical system, which spread across their empire.

- Ancient China: Traditional Chinese Medicine (TCM) has a rich history of herbalism, with the "Shennong Bencao Jing" (The Divine Farmer's Materia Medica) serving as a cornerstone text. This ancient pharmacopeia classified hundreds of herbs and their medicinal properties, laying the foundation for a holistic approach to healing that balances the body's energies.

- Ancient India: Ayurveda, meaning "science of life," is India's traditional system of medicine. It utilizes a vast array of herbal remedies to balance the body's doshas (energies) and promote wellness. The "Charaka Samhita" and "Sushruta Samhita" are key texts that detail herbal preparations and their therapeutic uses.

Medieval Herbalism: How Herbalism Evolved During the Middle Ages

The Middle Ages saw the continuation and expansion of herbal knowledge, with monasteries playing a pivotal role in the preservation and dissemination of this wisdom.

- Monasteries across Europe cultivated medicinal herb gardens, and monks compiled herbals—books that described the properties and uses of plants. These texts were among the first to be printed after the invention of the printing press, making herbal knowledge more widely accessible.

- In the Islamic world, scholars translated and expanded upon Greek and Roman texts, adding their observations and discoveries. The works of Avicenna, particularly "The Canon of Medicine," integrated herbal remedies into a comprehensive medical system that influenced both the Islamic world and medieval Europe.

Renaissance to Modern Times: The Transition of Herbalism

The Renaissance period ignited a renewed interest in the study of herbalism, with scholars revisiting and revising ancient texts. This era saw the publication of many herbals, including those by Paracelsus, who introduced the concept of using minerals and chemicals in medicine, and Nicholas Culpeper, who democratized herbal knowledge by writing in English rather than Latin.

- The Age of Exploration introduced Europeans to new plants and herbal remedies from the Americas, Africa, and Asia, expanding the herbal pharmacopeia.

- However, the rise of modern medicine in the 19th and 20th centuries, with its focus on synthetic drugs and surgical interventions, led to a decline in the use of herbal remedies in the West.

Despite this, the 20th and 21st centuries have witnessed a resurgence in interest in herbalism, fueled by a growing awareness of the limitations of conventional medicine and a desire for more natural and holistic approaches to health. This revival is supported by scientific research into the efficacy of herbal remedies and a global movement towards sustainability and biodiversity, recognizing the importance of preserving traditional knowledge and the natural world from which it springs.

The historical journey of herbal remedies is a testament to the enduring human belief in the healing power of plants. From ancient civilizations to the modern era, herbalism has evolved, adapted, and flourished, reflecting humanity's continuous quest for health and well-being through the natural world. As we move forward, the lessons of the past guide us in harnessing the potential of herbal remedies to address contemporary health challenges, ensuring that this ancient art remains a vital part of our collective heritage and future.

Herbal practiccs in Ancicnt Egypt, Greece, Rome, China, and India.

The profound relationship between humans and the plant kingdom is beautifully illustrated through the herbal practices of ancient civilizations. These practices, deeply embedded in the daily lives and spiritual beliefs of ancient societies, showcase the ingenuity and depth of knowledge our ancestors possessed regarding the medicinal properties of plants.

In Ancient Egypt, the use of medicinal plants was highly advanced. The Ebers Papyrus, dating back to around 1550 BCE, is one of the oldest and most significant medical documents from this era, listing over 850 herbal remedies. Egyptians utilized garlic to enhance heart health and aloe vera for its skin-healing properties. Herbs also played a vital role in their spiritual rituals, including the embalming process, demonstrating the intertwined nature of health, religion, and the afterlife in Egyptian culture.

The Greeks and Romans furthered the medicinal use of plants, integrating herbalism into the foundation of Western medicine. Hippocrates, often referred to as the father of medicine, emphasized the healing powers of nature and the importance of dietary and herbal treatments. Dioscorides, in his seminal work "De Materia Medica," cataloged over 600 plants, their uses, and their preparations, a text that remained a critical reference for over 1,500 years. Roman contributions included the expansion of the herbal compendium and the establishment of formal medical practices that incorporated these ancient herbal remedies.

In Ancient China, the holistic approach to health was embodied in Traditional Chinese Medicine (TCM), where herbalism played a crucial role. The "Shennong Bencao Jing" (The Divine Farmer's Materia Medica), compiled around the 1st century CE, classified hundreds of medicinal plants and minerals, emphasizing the balance of bodily energies (Qi) and the harmony between humans and their environment. This text laid the groundwork for a sophisticated system of medicine that integrates herbal remedies with acupuncture, massage, and dietary therapy.

Ancient India's Ayurvedic medicine is another testament to the sophisticated use of herbal remedies. Ayurveda, translating to "science of life," focuses on balancing the body's three doshas (vital energies) to maintain health. Foundational texts like the "Charaka Samhita" and the "Sushruta Samhita" detail the properties and uses of hundreds of plants, highlighting the importance of herbs in promoting physical, mental, and spiritual well-being.

These ancient civilizations, each with their unique approach to herbalism, contributed significantly to the global knowledge of plant-based medicine. Their practices, deeply rooted in observation, experimentation, and spiritual beliefs, laid the foundation for modern herbalism and continue to inspire contemporary practices. The legacy of these ancient herbalists, with their profound respect for nature and its healing powers, underscores the timeless relevance of herbal remedies in promoting health and wellness.

Medieval Herbalism

During the Middle Ages, herbalism flourished within the confines of monasteries and through the traditions of folk medicine, becoming a cornerstone of medical knowledge and practice. This period, extending roughly from the 5th to the 15th century, witnessed a significant evolution in the use of herbal remedies, shaped by the social, religious, and cultural landscapes of medieval Europe. Monastic medicine emerged as a pivotal force in the preservation and advancement of herbal knowledge. Monasteries, with their cloistered gardens, became sanctuaries for medicinal plants. Monks and nuns devoted themselves to the cultivation of herbs, drawing on ancient texts and local traditions to treat both their communities and the laypeople who sought their aid.

These religious communities were among the few literate segments of society, enabling them to study and transcribe ancient Greek, Roman, and Arabic works on herbalism, thereby preserving this invaluable knowledge through the Dark Ages.

• Herb Gardens and Apothecaries: Every monastery had its herb garden, or "physic garden," where plants were carefully cultivated for their healing properties. These gardens served as living libraries of medicinal plants, including sage, rosemary, thyme, and lavender, among others. Monks and nuns became adept at preparing a variety of herbal remedies, from simple teas and tinctures to complex salves and poultices.

• Herbal Manuscripts and Texts: Monastic scribes diligently copied and illustrated herbal manuscripts, which detailed the medicinal uses of plants. These texts, often adorned with meticulous illustrations, were instrumental in the transmission of herbal knowledge across Europe. The "Herbarius" and "Hortus Sanitatis" are notable examples of early printed herbals that drew extensively on monastic writings.

Folk remedies, deeply rooted in local traditions and the wisdom of healers, wise women, and herbalists, also played a crucial role in the practice of medieval herbalism. These remedies were passed down orally from generation to generation, reflecting a deep connection to the natural world and an intuitive understanding of the healing properties of plants.

• Local Knowledge and Practices: Folk herbalism thrived on the knowledge of local flora and the traditional practices of rural communities. Herbalists, often women, used their intimate knowledge of the land to gather wild herbs and prepare remedies for a wide range of ailments. This tradition was characterized by a holistic approach to healing, considering not only the physical symptoms but also the emotional and spiritual well-being of the patient.

• Community Healers: In villages and hamlets, the village healer or wise woman was a central figure, offering guidance and remedies for health issues. These practitioners often relied on a combination of herbs, charms, and rituals to treat their patients, embodying a holistic approach to health that integrated body, mind, and spirit. The synthesis of monastic and folk traditions during the Middle Ages laid the groundwork for the Renaissance of herbalism that followed. This period of history is marked by a rich tapestry of herbal knowledge, reflecting the diverse influences and practices that shaped the use of medicinal plants. The legacy of medieval herbalism is evident in the continued use of many traditional remedies and the enduring interest in natural, plant-based medicine. Through the diligent efforts of monks, nuns, and folk practitioners, the wisdom of the past was preserved, allowing future generations to benefit from the healing power of herbs.

The transition of herbalism through the Renaissance and its place in contemporary medicine.

The Renaissance marked a pivotal era in the evolution of herbalism, characterized by a profound revival of interest in the natural sciences and a re-examination of classical texts. This period saw the emergence of notable figures such as Paracelsus, who championed the use of chemicals in medicine, yet also emphasized the importance of plants. His doctrine, "The dose makes the poison," underscored the nuanced understanding of herbal remedies' potency and toxicity, laying foundational principles for pharmacology. Meanwhile, Nicholas Culpeper's translations of medical works into English democratized herbal knowledge, making it accessible to the layperson and not just the Latin-educated elite. Culpeper's herbal compendiums combined astrological insights with plant lore, illustrating the era's holistic approach to healing.

• Herbal Renaissance: The printing press's invention facilitated the widespread dissemination of herbal compendiums, significantly enhancing the public's access to knowledge about medicinal plants. This democratization of information contributed to an explosion of interest in herbal medicine across Europe.

• Global Expansion: The Age of Exploration expanded the European pharmacopeia by introducing new plants from the Americas, Asia, and Africa. This global exchange of botanical knowledge enriched herbal traditions, incorporating plants like tobacco, quinine, and cacao into European medicine, which had profound implications for both healing practices and the burgeoning field of botany.

As we transitioned into the modern era, the 19th and early 20th centuries witnessed a shift towards synthetic pharmaceuticals, with the isolation of active compounds from plants leading to the development of drugs such as aspirin, derived from willow bark. This period marked a decline in the traditional practice of herbalism in the West, as the scientific method and standardized medicine began to dominate.

However, the late 20th and early 21st centuries have seen a resurgence of interest in herbalism, driven by a growing disillusionment with the limitations and side effects of conventional medicine, as well as an increasing awareness of the importance of sustainability and natural wellness. This modern herbal renaissance is characterized by:

• Scientific Validation: Contemporary research has begun to validate the efficacy of many traditional herbal remedies, leading to a more integrative approach in which herbalism and conventional medicine complement each other. This synergy is evident in the rising popularity of phytotherapy, which applies scientific research to traditional herbal practices.

• Holistic Health Movement: The holistic health movement has embraced herbalism as a key component of wellness, emphasizing prevention over cure and the treatment of the whole person. This approach aligns with the increasing consumer desire for natural and organic products, including herbal supplements.

• Cultural Revival and Integration: There is a growing recognition of the value of indigenous and traditional herbal practices, leading to efforts to preserve this knowledge and integrate it into contemporary healthcare. This cultural revival also reflects a broader societal shift towards sustainability and environmental stewardship, with herbalism playing a role in the movement towards more sustainable healthcare practices.

• Regulation and Professionalization: The field of herbalism is becoming increasingly regulated and professionalized, with certifications and standards ensuring the quality and safety of herbal products. This development helps to bridge the gap between traditional herbalism and modern healthcare, ensuring that herbal remedies can be safely and effectively integrated into contemporary medical practices.

In conclusion, the journey of herbalism from the Renaissance to modern times reflects a dynamic interplay between tradition and innovation. As we continue to explore the potential of plants in healing and wellness, the lessons of the past inform our approach to integrating herbalism into contemporary medicine, offering a more holistic, sustainable, and personalized approach to health.

CHAPTER 3: UNDERSTANDING PLANTS AND THEIR PROPERTIES

Botanical Basics: An introduction to botany for herbalists begins with recognizing the immense diversity within the plant kingdom. Plants, from towering trees to modest herbs, possess a complex structure that serves both their survival and medicinal properties. Understanding the anatomy of plants is crucial for herbalists, as different parts of a plant—roots, stems, leaves, flowers, and seeds—contain unique compounds beneficial for health.

• Roots often store a concentration of powerful compounds. They anchor the plant, absorb water and nutrients, and can be potent in remedies for their grounding and nourishing properties.

• Stems provide support, allowing the plant to grow towards the light. They transport fluids between the roots and leaves. The stem's makeup, whether woody or soft, can influence its use in herbal preparations.

• Leaves are the primary site of photosynthesis, converting sunlight into energy. They can be rich in healing compounds and are often used in teas, tinctures, and topical applications.

• Flowers are the reproductive parts of the plant and can contain essential oils and other compounds beneficial for health. They are frequently used in remedies for their potent aromatic and therapeutic properties.

• Seeds are the plant's future, carrying the genetic blueprint and often concentrated nutrients and compounds. They can be used in herbal medicine for their restorative properties.

Phytochemistry: The chemical compounds in plants, known as phytochemicals, are the basis for their medicinal properties. These compounds can act as antioxidants, anti-inflammatories, antivirals, and more, contributing to the plant's ability to protect itself from pests and diseases. For humans, these compounds can offer similar protective and healing benefits. Key phytochemicals include alkaloids, flavonoids, tannins, and terpenes.

• Alkaloids have pronounced effects on the human body and can be found in plants like belladonna and echinacea. They are known for their analgesic and antibacterial properties.

• Flavonoids are known for their antioxidant and anti-inflammatory effects, found in a wide range of plants, including berries and green tea.

• Tannins, present in plants like witch hazel, have astringent properties, making them useful in treating wounds and inflammation.

• Terpenes contribute to the aromatic qualities of plants and have a variety of therapeutic effects. Lavender, for example, contains linalool, a terpene known for its calming and anti-anxiety properties.

Harvesting and Sustainability: Responsible harvesting practices ensure the longevity and health of plant populations and their surrounding ecosystems. Overharvesting and habitat destruction pose significant threats to the availability of medicinal plants. Herbalists must prioritize sustainability by:

• Harvesting in a manner that allows plants to regenerate, taking only what is needed and leaving enough for the plant to continue its growth cycle.

• Identifying and using abundant plants instead of those that are rare or endangered. Cultivating medicinal herbs in gardens or containers can reduce pressure on wild populations.

• Understanding the best times to harvest different parts of the plant for optimal potency. For example, leaves are often most vibrant just before flowering, while roots may be harvested in the fall when the plant's energy is stored below ground.

• Practicing ethical wildcrafting, which includes obtaining permission to harvest on private land, respecting local and indigenous knowledge, and avoiding areas exposed to pollutants or pesticides.

By integrating these principles, herbalists can deepen their connection to the natural world, ensuring that the practice of herbalism remains a sustainable and healing art for generations to come.

Botanical Basics

Understanding the foundational elements of botany is essential for any herbalist. This knowledge not only enriches one's appreciation of the plant world but also enhances the ability to select and utilize herbs more effectively for medicinal purposes. The study of botany for herbalists encompasses several key areas, including plant taxonomy, anatomy, life cycles, and ecology, each offering insights into how plants grow, reproduce, and interact with their environment.

Plant Taxonomy is the science of naming, describing, and classifying plants. It provides a universal language for herbalists, enabling them to identify plants accurately and understand their relationships. Plants are categorized into families, genera, and species, with each level providing specific information about their characteristics and uses. For instance, members of the Mint family (Lamiaceae) are known for their aromatic properties and include familiar herbs such as basil, lavender, and mint.

Anatomy of Plants delves into the structure of plants, highlighting the parts that are most often used in herbal medicine:

- Roots, such as those of the dandelion, are often used for their detoxifying properties.

- Stems, like those of the licorice plant, can support the respiratory system.

- Leaves, from plants like peppermint, are widely used for their digestive benefits.

- Flowers, such as chamomile, are cherished for their calming effects.

- Seeds, including fennel, are utilized for their ability to soothe digestive discomfort.

Understanding the specific functions and benefits of each plant part can guide herbalists in selecting the right form of the herb for their remedies.

Life Cycles of Plants are crucial for understanding when to harvest. Annual plants complete their life cycle in one year, biennials in two, and perennials live for multiple years. Harvesting at the right time in a plant's life cycle ensures the highest concentration of active constituents. For example, harvesting roots in the fall when perennial plants have stored nutrients in their roots for the winter can yield a more potent medicine.

Ecology examines the relationship between plants and their environment. It includes understanding the specific conditions under which plants thrive, such as soil type, climate, and interactions with other plants and animals. This knowledge is vital for sustainable harvesting and cultivation practices, ensuring that herbalists can grow or wildcraft herbs without harming the ecosystem.

Sustainability and Ethical Wildcrafting practices are integral to botanical basics. Herbalists must be stewards of the land, harvesting in ways that do not deplete natural resources or harm plant populations. This includes:

- Taking only what is needed and leaving enough behind for the plant to regenerate.

- Harvesting in a way that does not disturb the surrounding environment or wildlife.

- Using parts of the plant that regenerate quickly, such as leaves, rather than those that are slow to grow, like roots.

By grounding themselves in the basics of botany, herbalists gain a deeper understanding and respect for the plants they work with. This foundation not only enhances the effectiveness of their remedies but also contributes to the preservation of herbal traditions and the health of the planet.

Phytochemistry

Phytochemistry explores the fascinating world of chemical compounds in plants, known as phytochemicals, which are responsible for their medicinal properties. These natural compounds play a crucial role in the plant's defense mechanisms against predators, diseases, and environmental stress, and when used in herbal medicine, they can offer significant health benefits to humans.

Phytochemicals are categorized into several major groups, each with unique properties and health effects:

- Alkaloids: These nitrogen-containing compounds are found in plants such as belladonna (Atropa belladonna), goldenseal (Hydrastis canadensis), and echinacea (Echinacea spp.). Alkaloids have a wide range of pharmacological activities, including analgesic (pain relief), antibacterial, and anti-inflammatory effects. For example, morphine, an alkaloid derived from the opium poppy (Papaver somniferum), is a potent analgesic used in modern medicine.

- Flavonoids: This diverse group of phytochemicals is known for its antioxidant and anti-inflammatory properties. Flavonoids are abundant in fruits, vegetables, tea, and wine. They help protect against chronic diseases such as heart disease and cancer by scavenging harmful free radicals in the body. Quercetin, a flavonoid found in onions (Allium cepa), apples (Malus domestica), and berries, is particularly noted for its anti-inflammatory and antihistamine effects.

- Tannins: These polyphenolic compounds are present in a wide variety of plants, including witch hazel (Hamamelis virginiana) and oak bark (Quercus spp.). Tannins have astringent properties, which make them effective in treating wounds and inflammation. They can help reduce swelling and speed up the healing process by precipitating proteins and protecting the affected area from infection.

- Terpenes and Terpenoids: Terpenes are the primary constituents of essential oils derived from plants such as lavender (Lavandula angustifolia) and rosemary (Rosmarinus officinalis). They are responsible for the aromatic qualities of plants and have a variety of therapeutic effects, including anti-anxiety, anti-inflammatory, and analgesic properties. Linalool, a terpene found in lavender, is well-known for its calming and sleep-inducing effects.

- Glycosides: These compounds consist of a sugar molecule bonded to a non-sugar molecule and are found in plants like foxglove (Digitalis purpurea) and senna (Senna alexandrina). Glycosides have diverse health effects, including cardiac stimulation and laxative properties. For example, digoxin, derived from foxglove, is a powerful glycoside used to treat heart failure. Understanding the phytochemistry of medicinal plants is essential for herbalists and practitioners of natural medicine, as it provides a scientific basis for the therapeutic use of herbs. By identifying the active compounds in herbs and understanding their effects on the human body, herbalists can more effectively formulate remedies for a wide range of conditions.

Moreover, the study of phytochemistry highlights the importance of preserving biodiversity and natural habitats. Many phytochemicals have yet to be discovered, and the loss of plant species could mean the loss of potential medicinal compounds. Sustainable harvesting and conservation efforts are crucial to ensure that these natural resources remain available for future generations. Incorporating phytochemical knowledge into herbal practice not only enhances the efficacy of herbal remedies but also deepens our appreciation for the complexity and richness of the plant kingdom. As research in phytochemistry advances, it continues to unlock the healing potential of plants, bridging the gap between traditional herbalism and modern science.

Harvesting and Sustainability

Harvesting and using herbs responsibly is a cornerstone of sustainable herbalism. This practice not only ensures the longevity of plant species but also respects the ecosystems where these plants grow. Here, we delve into the principles of ethical harvesting and sustainable use of herbs, providing a guide for both novice and experienced herbalists.

Ethical Harvesting Practices

• Seek Permission: Before harvesting wild herbs, it's crucial to seek permission from the landowner or governing body, especially in protected areas.

• Sustainable Harvesting Techniques: Always use clean, sharp tools to make precise cuts, which help plants recover quickly. Harvest no more than one-third of a plant or patch to ensure it can continue to grow and propagate.

• Timing Matters: Harvest herbs at the right time of day and season to ensure the highest potency. Generally, the best time is in the morning after the dew has dried but before the sun is too intense.

• Leave No Trace: Be mindful of your impact on the environment. Avoid trampling surrounding plants and ensure you leave the area as you found it.

Sustainable Use of Herbs

• Cultivate Your Own: Whenever possible, grow your own herbs. This not only reduces pressure on wild populations but also gives you control over the growing conditions, ensuring they are free from harmful chemicals.

• Source Responsibly: When purchasing herbs, choose suppliers who prioritize sustainability and ethical harvesting practices. Look for certifications that indicate organic and fair-trade practices.

• Use Every Part: Make the most of the herbs you harvest or purchase by using all parts of the plant. Roots, stems, leaves, flowers, and seeds can all have valuable medicinal properties.

• Composting: Return unused plant materials to the earth through composting. This practice supports soil health and contributes to a cycle of growth and renewal.

Conservation Efforts

• Support Conservation Organizations: Engage with and support organizations working to protect plant biodiversity and promote sustainable herbalism practices.

• Educate Others: Share your knowledge of sustainable harvesting and use of herbs with your community. Education is a powerful tool in the conservation of herbal medicine traditions.

• Participate in Plant Rescue Operations: In areas undergoing development, participate in efforts to rescue and relocate native plants to safe environments where they can thrive.

Final Thoughts

Adopting sustainable and ethical practices in harvesting and using herbs is not only an act of respect towards nature but also a step towards ensuring the availability of medicinal plants for future generations. By integrating these practices into our daily lives, we contribute to the health of our planet and continue the ancient tradition of herbalism in a responsible and conscious manner.

CHAPTER 4: COMMON MEDICINAL HERBS AND THEIR USES

Herbs for Common Ailments

The natural world offers a bounty of medicinal herbs that have been used for centuries to treat common ailments. These plants contain compounds that can support health and wellness, often with fewer side effects than conventional medications. Here, we explore some of the most widely used medicinal herbs and their applications.

Echinacea (Echinacea spp.)

• Uses: Known for its immune-boosting properties, Echinacea is commonly used to prevent or treat colds and respiratory infections.

• Preparation: Often consumed as tea, tinctures, or capsules.

• Safety Rating: ♥♥♥♥♡ Generally safe, but consult a healthcare provider if you have autoimmune diseases.

Ginger (Zingiber officinale)

• Uses: Ginger is revered for its anti-inflammatory and anti-nausea effects, making it a go-to remedy for digestive issues, morning sickness, and motion sickness.

• Preparation: Can be used fresh, dried, or as an extract in teas, foods, and supplements.

• Safety Rating: ♥♥♥♥♡ Safe for most people; excessive consumption can cause heartburn or irritation.

Turmeric (Curcuma longa)

• Uses: Contains curcumin, known for its potent anti-inflammatory and antioxidant properties. Useful in managing arthritis pain and enhancing overall health.

• Preparation: Added to foods, teas, or taken as supplements for concentrated doses.

• Safety Rating: ♥♥♥♡♡ Consult with a healthcare provider before using high-dose supplements, especially if on blood thinners.

Peppermint (Mentha piperita)

• Uses: Peppermint oil is effective in relieving digestive symptoms, such as irritable bowel syndrome (IBS), nausea, and indigestion.

• Preparation: Consumed as tea, capsules, or essential oil (for topical use).

• Safety Rating: ♥♥♥♥♡ Peppermint leaf is generally safe; peppermint oil should be used cautiously as it can cause heartburn or allergic reactions.

Lavender (Lavandula angustifolia)

• Uses: Known for its calming and sleep-inducing effects, lavender is used to reduce anxiety, improve sleep, and alleviate stress.

• Preparation: Used in aromatherapy, teas, or topical applications.

• Safety Rating: ♥♥♥♥♡ Generally safe; avoid oral consumption of essential oil without professional guidance.

Chamomile (Matricaria chamomilla)

• Uses: Chamomile is widely recognized for its calming effects, making it a popular choice for treating insomnia, anxiety, and digestive upset.

• Preparation: Most commonly consumed as tea; also available in topical and oral forms.

• Safety Rating: ♥♥♥♥♡ Well tolerated; rare allergic reactions in individuals sensitive to the Asteraceae family.

Garlic (Allium sativum)

• Uses: Garlic has cardiovascular benefits, including lowering blood pressure and cholesterol levels. It also has antimicrobial properties.

• Preparation: Can be eaten raw, cooked, or taken as supplements.

• Safety Rating: ❤❤❤♡♡ Safe for most; may interact with blood thinners and cause digestive discomfort in some.

Superfoods and Adaptogens

Beyond treating specific ailments, certain herbs are celebrated for their overall health-enhancing properties. These "superfoods" and adaptogens support the body's ability to resist stressors, improve energy levels, and boost immunity.

Ashwagandha (Withania somnifera)

• Uses: An adaptogen that helps the body manage stress, improves energy levels, and supports overall well-being.

• Preparation: Available in powders, capsules, and tinctures.

• Safety Rating: ❤❤❤♡♡ Consult a healthcare provider before use, especially if pregnant, nursing, or on medication.

Spirulina (Arthrospira platensis)

• Uses: A nutrient-rich blue-green algae considered a superfood, spirulina is packed with vitamins, minerals, and antioxidants.

• Preparation: Available in tablets, powders, and flakes to add to smoothies and foods.

• Safety Rating: ❤❤❤❤♡ Generally safe; source from reputable suppliers to avoid contaminants.

Ginseng (Panax ginseng)

• Uses: An adaptogen that enhances mental clarity, energy levels, and immune function.

• Preparation: Consumed as tea, in capsules, or as a liquid extract.

• Safety Rating: ❤❤❤♡♡ May interact with certain medications and is not recommended for individuals with hormone-sensitive conditions.

Incorporating these herbs into your daily routine can offer a natural way to support your health and well-being. However, it's important to consult with a healthcare provider before starting any new herbal regimen, especially if you have existing health conditions or are taking medications.

By understanding the uses, preparations, and safety considerations of these common medicinal herbs, you can make informed choices about incorporating herbal remedies into your life.

Herbs for Common Ailments

Echinacea (Echinacea spp.)

Echinacea stands out for its remarkable immune-enhancing properties, making it a first-line defense against colds and upper respiratory infections. The active compounds within Echinacea help stimulate the immune system, potentially reducing the duration and severity of symptoms.

• Preparation: Echinacea can be consumed in various forms, including teas, capsules, and tinctures. For cold prevention, starting doses at the first sign of symptoms is recommended.

• Dosage: Follow manufacturer's instructions for supplements. For tea, steep 1-2 teaspoons of dried herb in hot water for 10-15 minutes, up to three times daily.

• Safety Considerations: Generally well-tolerated; some individuals may experience mild side effects like dizziness or rash. Those with autoimmune diseases should consult a healthcare provider before use.

Ginger (Zingiber officinale)

Ginger's potent anti-inflammatory and antioxidative properties make it an effective remedy for a wide range of digestive issues, including nausea, indigestion, and motion sickness. Its warming effect is also beneficial in treating colds and flu by promoting sweating and expelling warmth.

• Preparation: Fresh ginger root can be used in cooking or made into tea. Ginger supplements are available for those who prefer a more concentrated form.

• Dosage: For tea, use about one-half teaspoon of grated ginger per cup of hot water. Supplements should be taken according to the package directions.

• Safety Considerations: Ginger is safe for most people, but high doses may lead to heartburn or digestive discomfort. Pregnant women should limit intake to avoid potential effects on fetal sex hormones.

Turmeric (Curcuma longa)

Turmeric, with its active component curcumin, offers powerful anti-inflammatory benefits, making it effective in managing conditions like arthritis and other inflammatory disorders. Its antioxidant properties also contribute to overall health and wellness.

• Preparation: Incorporate turmeric into meals or take as a supplement for a more concentrated dose. Turmeric tea is another enjoyable way to consume this herb.

• Dosage: When using in cooking, there's no specific limit, though one should be mindful of the strong flavor. Supplemental doses typically range from 500-2,000 mg of curcumin per day.

• Safety Considerations: Turmeric is generally safe; however, high doses or long-term use can cause gastrointestinal issues. Consult a healthcare provider before use, especially if taking blood thinners.

Peppermint (Mentha piperita)

Peppermint is renowned for its soothing effect on the digestive system, offering relief from symptoms of IBS, nausea, and indigestion. The menthol in peppermint helps relax the muscles of the digestive tract, easing discomfort.

• Preparation: Peppermint tea is a popular and effective way to enjoy its benefits. Peppermint oil capsules are also available for more targeted digestive support.

• Dosage: For tea, steep 1 teaspoon of dried peppermint leaves in hot water for 10 minutes. Peppermint oil capsules should be taken as directed on the package.

• Safety Considerations: While peppermint leaf is safe for most, peppermint oil should be used with caution as it can cause heartburn or allergic reactions in some individuals.

Lavender (Lavandula angustifolia)

Lavender is widely appreciated for its calming and sedative properties, making it an excellent herb for reducing anxiety, improving sleep quality, and managing stress. Its gentle action makes it suitable for regular use.

• Preparation: Lavender can be used in aromatherapy, added to baths, or brewed as tea. Lavender oil can be applied topically or diffused for inhalation.

• Dosage: For tea, use 1-2 teaspoons of dried lavender flowers per cup of boiling water. In aromatherapy, a few drops of oil can be used as needed.

• Safety Considerations: Lavender is generally safe; however, oral ingestion of the essential oil should be avoided unless under professional guidance.

Chamomile (Matricaria chamomilla)

Chamomile is a gentle, soothing herb, ideal for addressing insomnia, anxiety, and mild digestive issues. Its anti-inflammatory properties also make it useful for skin conditions when applied topically.

• Preparation: Chamomile tea is the most common form of consumption, providing a calming effect. It can also be used in creams or ointments for topical application.

• Dosage: For tea, steep 2-3 teaspoons of dried chamomile flowers in hot water for 10 minutes. Drink 1-3 times daily or before bedtime for sleep support.

• Safety Considerations: Chamomile is well-tolerated by most, but those with allergies to plants in the Asteraceae family should proceed with caution.

Incorporating these herbs into your health regimen can offer natural, effective relief for common ailments. Always consult with a healthcare provider before beginning any new herbal treatment, especially if you have existing health conditions or are taking other medications.

Superfoods and Adaptogens

Superfoods and adaptogens represent a category of herbs and plants that are not just beneficial for treating specific ailments but are pivotal in enhancing overall health, vitality, and resilience against stress. These powerful botanicals are packed with nutrients and compounds that support the body's natural ability to balance and heal itself. Here, we delve into some of the most potent superfoods and adaptogens, exploring their health benefits and how to incorporate them into your daily regimen.

Ashwagandha (Withania somnifera)

Ashwagandha, a cornerstone herb in Ayurvedic medicine, is renowned for its adaptogenic properties. It aids the body in managing stress by modulating the release of stress hormones. It's also known for improving sleep quality, enhancing energy levels, and supporting cognitive function.

- Preparation: Ashwagandha can be taken in powder form, mixed into beverages or smoothies, or as capsules and tinctures for a more concentrated dose.

- Dosage: Typical dosages range from 300 to 500 mg of extract daily, though it's advisable to start with lower doses to assess tolerance.

- Safety Rating: ♥♥♥♡♡. While generally safe, it's recommended to consult with a healthcare provider before starting, especially for pregnant or nursing women.

Spirulina (Arthrospira platensis)

Spirulina, a blue-green algae, is a nutrient-dense superfood. It's an excellent source of protein, vitamins B1, B2, and B3, copper, iron, magnesium, potassium, and manganese. Spirulina also contains powerful antioxidants and has been shown to have anti-inflammatory effects.

- Preparation: Available in tablets, powders, and flakes, spirulina can be easily added to smoothies, juices, or sprinkled on salads and dishes.

- Dosage: A standard dose can range from 1 to 3 grams per day, but it's safe to consume up to 10 grams daily.

- Safety Rating: ♥♥♥♥♡. Ensure sourcing from reputable suppliers to avoid contamination with heavy metals or harmful bacteria.

Ginseng (Panax ginseng)

Ginseng is an adaptogen famed for its ability to enhance mental performance, boost energy levels, and support immune function. It has been used in traditional Chinese medicine for centuries to combat fatigue and strengthen the body's stress response.

- Preparation: Ginseng can be consumed as tea, in capsules, or as a liquid extract. Fresh or dried ginseng root can also be chewed or added to recipes.

- Dosage: Recommended dosages vary, but a general guideline is 200 to 400 mg of extract daily.

- Safety Rating: ♥♥♥♡♡. Ginseng may interact with certain medications and is not recommended for individuals with hormone-sensitive conditions.

Maca (Lepidium meyenii)

Maca root, often referred to as Peruvian ginseng, is a cruciferous vegetable native to Peru. It's known for its ability to enhance strength, stamina, and libido. Maca is also rich in vitamins, minerals, and plant sterols that can improve mood and energy.

- Preparation: Maca powder can be added to smoothies, oatmeal, or baked goods. It's also available in capsules for those who prefer not to taste it.

- Dosage: A typical dosage ranges from 1.5 to 5 grams per day.

- Safety Rating: ❤❤❤❤♡. Maca is considered safe for most people, but its effects on hormone-sensitive conditions are not well understood.

Matcha (Camellia sinensis)

Matcha is a type of green tea that comes in a powdered form and is known for its high concentration of antioxidants, particularly EGCG (epigallocatechin gallate), which has been linked to numerous health benefits, including reduced risk of heart disease and certain cancers, as well as improved brain function.

- Preparation: Matcha powder can be whisked into hot water to make tea, blended into smoothies, or used in cooking and baking.

- Dosage: For health benefits, consuming 1 to 2 teaspoons of matcha powder per day is recommended.

- Safety Rating: ❤❤❤❤♡. Matcha is safe for most people, but due to its caffeine content, those sensitive to caffeine should consume it in moderation.

Incorporating these superfoods and adaptogens into your daily routine can significantly contribute to your overall health and well-being.

They offer a natural way to enhance your body's resilience to stress, boost energy levels, and support a healthy immune system. However, always consult with a healthcare provider before introducing any new supplements into your diet, especially if you have existing health conditions or are taking medications.

CHAPTER 5: HERBAL REMEDIES FOR SPECIFIC HEALTH CONDITIONS

Respiratory Health

Herbs have been used for centuries to support respiratory health, offering relief from symptoms of colds, flu, asthma, and allergies. These natural remedies can soothe irritation, reduce inflammation, and enhance the body's immune response.

Eucalyptus (Eucalyptus globulus)

- Uses: Eucalyptus leaves contain eucalyptol, a compound that helps break up mucus and relieve congestion. It's also known for its antimicrobial properties, making it beneficial in treating respiratory infections.

- Preparation: Inhalation of eucalyptus steam by adding a few drops of eucalyptus oil to hot water or using a diffuser. Eucalyptus leaves can also be used to make tea.

- Dosage: For steam inhalation, use 2-3 drops of eucalyptus oil in hot water. For tea, steep 1-2 teaspoons of dried leaves in boiling water for 10 minutes.

- Safety Considerations: Eucalyptus oil should not be ingested or applied undiluted to the skin. Pregnant and breastfeeding women should avoid its use.

Mullein (Verbascum thapsus)

- Uses: Mullein is traditionally used for its ability to soothe the respiratory tract and reduce inflammation. It's particularly effective in treating dry coughs and bronchitis.

- Preparation: Mullein leaves and flowers can be used to prepare tea. Mullein oil is also used for ear infections.

- Dosage: For tea, steep 1-2 teaspoons of dried mullein leaves or flowers in boiling water for 10-15 minutes. Drink up to 3 cups daily.

- Safety Considerations: Generally safe, but some individuals may experience allergic reactions. Always strain tea to remove fine hairs that can irritate the throat.

Digestive Health

Herbal remedies can provide significant relief for various digestive disorders, including indigestion, IBS, and other gastrointestinal issues, by soothing the digestive tract, reducing inflammation, and promoting healthy gut flora.

Peppermint (Mentha piperita)

- Uses: Peppermint is effective in relieving symptoms of IBS, such as cramping and bloating. Its antispasmodic properties help relax the muscles of the digestive tract.

- Preparation: Peppermint tea or enteric-coated peppermint oil capsules.

- Dosage: For tea, steep 1 teaspoon of dried peppermint leaves in hot water for 10 minutes. If using capsules, follow the manufacturer's instructions.

- Safety Considerations: Peppermint oil capsules should not be used by individuals with GERD as it may worsen symptoms.

Ginger (Zingiber officinale)

- Uses: Ginger is renowned for its anti-nausea and anti-inflammatory effects, making it a go-to remedy for motion sickness, morning sickness, and digestive discomfort.

- Preparation: Fresh ginger root can be used in cooking, made into tea, or taken as supplements.

- Dosage: For tea, use one-half teaspoon of grated ginger per cup of hot water. Supplements should be taken according to package directions.

- Safety Considerations: Generally safe, but high doses may lead to heartburn or digestive discomfort. Pregnant women should consult a healthcare provider before use.

Mental Health

Herbs can play a supportive role in managing stress, anxiety, and sleep disorders, offering a natural way to enhance mental well-being and emotional balance.

Lavender (Lavandula angustifolia)

- Uses: Lavender is widely used for its calming and sedative properties, effective in reducing anxiety, improving sleep quality, and alleviating stress.

- Preparation: Aromatherapy using lavender oil, lavender tea, or capsules.

- Dosage: For aromatherapy, use a few drops of oil in a diffuser. For tea, steep 1-2 teaspoons of dried flowers in boiling water for 10 minutes.

- Safety Considerations: Generally safe; however, oral ingestion of the essential oil should be avoided unless under professional guidance.

Chamomile (Matricaria chamomilla)

- Uses: Chamomile is known for its gentle, soothing effect, making it ideal for treating insomnia and anxiety.

- Preparation: Chamomile tea or capsules.

- Dosage: For tea, steep 2-3 teaspoons of dried chamomile flowers in hot water for 10 minutes. Drink before bedtime for sleep support.

- Safety Considerations: Well-tolerated by most, but those with allergies to plants in the Asteraceae family should proceed with caution.

Skin Conditions

Natural treatments for skin conditions such as acne, eczema, and psoriasis can reduce inflammation, soothe irritation, and promote healing.

Aloe Vera (Aloe barbadensis miller)

- Uses: Aloe vera is renowned for its soothing, moisturizing, and healing properties, making it effective in treating burns, sunburns, and skin irritations.

- Preparation: Aloe vera gel can be applied directly to the affected area.

- Dosage: Apply a thin layer of gel to the skin as needed.

- Safety Considerations: Generally safe when applied topically. Oral consumption of aloe vera should be done cautiously as it can have laxative effects.

Calendula (Calendula officinalis)

- Uses: Calendula is used for its anti-inflammatory and healing properties, beneficial in treating eczema, psoriasis, and diaper rash.

- Preparation: Calendula cream, ointment, or infused oil can be applied to the skin.

- Dosage: Apply to the affected area 2-3 times daily.

- Safety Considerations: Generally safe; however, individuals allergic to plants in the Asteraceae family should test a small area first.

Women's Health

Herbal remedies offer natural support for menstruation, menopause, and reproductive health, addressing symptoms like cramps, hormonal imbalances, and hot flashes.

Black Cohosh (Actaea racemosa)

- Uses: Black cohosh is widely used for relieving menopause symptoms, including hot flashes, mood swings, and sleep disturbances.

- Preparation: Available in capsules, tinctures, or tea.

- Dosage: Follow manufacturer's instructions for capsules and tinctures. For tea, steep 1 teaspoon of dried root in boiling water for 20-30 minutes.

- Safety Considerations: Generally safe for short-term use. Pregnant or breastfeeding women should avoid it.

Chaste Tree Berry (Vitex agnus-castus)

- Uses: Chaste tree berry is beneficial in regulating menstrual cycles and easing PMS symptoms.

- Preparation: Available in capsules, tinctures, or tea.

- Dosage: Follow manufacturer's instructions for capsules and tinctures. For tea, steep 1 teaspoon of dried berries in boiling water for 10 minutes.

- Safety Considerations: Generally safe, but consult a healthcare provider before use, especially if pregnant, breastfeeding, or using hormonal medications.

By incorporating these herbal remedies into your health care regimen, you can harness the power of nature to address specific health conditions. Always consult with a healthcare provider before starting any new herbal treatment, especially if you have existing health conditions or are taking other medications.

Respiratory Health

Eucalyptus (Eucalyptus globulus) is a powerhouse for respiratory health, thanks to its main component, eucalyptol, which aids in breaking up mucus and clearing congestion. Its antimicrobial properties also make it a strong ally against respiratory infections. For a soothing inhalation, add 2-3 drops of eucalyptus oil to hot water and breathe in the steam, or use a diffuser to disperse its benefits throughout your environment. When preparing tea, steep 1-2 teaspoons of dried eucalyptus leaves in boiling water for 10 minutes. However, it's crucial to remember that eucalyptus oil should not be ingested or applied undiluted to the skin, and its use is not recommended for pregnant and breastfeeding women.

Mullein (Verbascum thapsus) stands out for its gentle action on the respiratory system, effectively soothing irritation and reducing inflammation. This herb is particularly beneficial for dry coughs and bronchitis. To harness its benefits, use mullein leaves and flowers to prepare tea by steeping 1-2 teaspoons in boiling water for 10-15

41

minutes. Drinking up to 3 cups daily can provide relief. Mullein oil, derived from the flowers, is also used for ear infections. It's generally safe for most people, but as with any herb, it's wise to strain the tea to remove fine hairs that could irritate the throat, and be aware of potential allergic reactions.

Thyme (Thymus vulgaris) is not only a culinary staple but also a potent herbal remedy for respiratory conditions, including bronchitis and coughs. Its natural antispasmodic and antibacterial properties make it an excellent choice for soothing coughs and fighting infections. For a simple thyme tea, steep 1-2 teaspoons of dried thyme in boiling water for 10 minutes. This tea can be consumed 2-3 times daily. Thyme is also beneficial as an inhalant; add a few drops of thyme essential oil to hot water for steam inhalation or use in a diffuser.

Licorice Root (Glycyrrhiza glabra) offers remarkable soothing and anti-inflammatory benefits, making it a go-to herb for conditions like sore throat and cough. Its demulcent properties help to soothe mucous membranes in the throat. Prepare licorice root tea by steeping 1 teaspoon of the dried root in boiling water for 10 minutes, and drink up to 2 cups daily. However, licorice root should be used with caution, especially for those with high blood pressure, heart disease, or pregnant women, due to its potential to affect blood pressure and potassium levels.

Marshmallow Root (Althaea officinalis) is another herb known for its demulcent properties, which provide a protective layer on the throat's mucous membranes, offering relief from coughs and sore throats. To make marshmallow root tea, steep 1-2 teaspoons of the dried root in cold water for several hours, then strain and drink. This cold infusion method helps to draw out the mucilaginous properties, providing maximum benefit.

Incorporating these herbs into your health care regimen can offer effective, natural relief for a variety of respiratory conditions. Always consult with a healthcare provider before starting any new herbal treatment, especially if you have existing health conditions or are taking other medications, to ensure safe and appropriate use.

Digestive Health

Digestive disorders, ranging from occasional indigestion to chronic conditions like Irritable Bowel Syndrome (IBS), affect millions of people worldwide. Fortunately, herbal remedies offer gentle yet effective ways to enhance digestive health and alleviate discomfort. By harnessing the power of specific herbs, individuals can support their digestive system naturally.

Peppermint (Mentha piperita)

Peppermint is renowned for its soothing effect on the gastrointestinal tract. Its antispasmodic properties help relax the muscles of the digestive system, making it an excellent remedy for indigestion and IBS symptoms such as cramping and bloating.

- Preparation: Peppermint tea is a popular and easy way to enjoy its benefits. Alternatively, enteric-coated peppermint oil capsules provide targeted relief for IBS symptoms.

- Dosage: For tea, steep 1 teaspoon of dried peppermint leaves in hot water for 10 minutes. If using capsules, follow the manufacturer's instructions, typically 1-2 capsules taken 2-3 times daily.

- Safety Considerations: While peppermint is generally safe, it may worsen symptoms of GERD (gastroesophageal reflux disease) due to relaxation of the esophageal sphincter.

Ginger (Zingiber officinale)

Ginger has been used for centuries to combat nausea, vomiting, and indigestion. Its natural anti-inflammatory and antiemetic properties make it a go-to remedy for motion sickness, morning sickness, and post-operative nausea.

- Preparation: Fresh ginger root can be steeped in hot water to make tea, added to meals, or chewed raw. Ginger supplements are also available for those who prefer a more concentrated form.

- Dosage: For tea, use about one-half teaspoon of grated ginger per cup of hot water. Supplements should be taken according to package directions, usually 250 mg 3-4 times daily.

- Safety Considerations: Ginger is safe for most people, but high doses may cause heartburn or digestive discomfort. Pregnant women should consult a healthcare provider due to potential effects on fetal sex hormones.

Fennel (Foeniculum vulgare)

Fennel seeds are effective in treating indigestion, bloating, and gas. They possess antispasmodic properties that can help relax the digestive tract muscles and alleviate discomfort.

- Preparation: Fennel tea can be made by steeping 1-2 teaspoons of crushed fennel seeds in boiling water. Fennel can also be chewed raw after meals to aid digestion.

- Dosage: Drink fennel tea up to three times daily or chew on half a teaspoon of fennel seeds post-meal.

- Safety Considerations: Fennel is generally safe, but pregnant women should use it cautiously as it has estrogenic effects.

Slippery Elm (Ulmus rubra)

Slippery elm contains mucilage, a substance that becomes a slick gel when mixed with water. This gel coats and soothes the mouth, throat, stomach, and intestines, making it beneficial for treating gastrointestinal irritation and conditions like GERD, IBS, and ulcerative colitis.

- Preparation: To make slippery elm tea, mix 1 tablespoon of powdered bark with hot water. Slippery elm capsules and lozenges are also available.

- Dosage: For tea, drink up to 3 cups daily. Follow manufacturer's instructions for capsules or lozenges.

- Safety Considerations: Slippery elm is considered safe, but because it can slow the absorption of medications, take it several hours before or after other medications.

Aloe Vera (Aloe barbadensis miller)

Aloe vera juice is known for its soothing properties on the digestive tract, helping to relieve constipation, soothe IBS symptoms, and reduce inflammation.

- Preparation: Aloe vera juice is available commercially. Ensure it is decolorized and purified for internal use.

- Dosage: Drink 1/4 to 1/2 cup of aloe vera juice daily, preferably on an empty stomach.

- Safety Considerations: Aloe vera juice should be used with caution as it can have a laxative effect. Avoid aloe preparations with aloin, which can be harsh on the digestive system.

Incorporating these herbal remedies into your daily routine can offer significant relief from digestive disorders. Always start with small doses to see how your body reacts and consult with a healthcare provider before using herbal treatments, especially if you have existing health conditions or are taking other medications.

Mental Health

Herbs have long been recognized for their ability to nurture mental well-being, offering natural remedies to reduce stress, alleviate anxiety, and promote restful sleep. In a world where mental health concerns are increasingly prevalent, turning to these natural allies can provide gentle, yet effective support for emotional balance and tranquility.

Herbs for Stress and Anxiety

• Ashwagandha (Withania somnifera): This adaptogen helps the body manage stress by reducing cortisol levels and modulating the stress response system.

  - Preparation: Ashwagandha can be taken as a powder mixed into beverages or food, or as capsules.

  - Dosage: A typical dosage is 300 to 500 mg of extract daily, though starting with a lower dose to assess tolerance is advisable.

  - Safety Rating: ♥♥♥♡♡. Consult a healthcare provider before use, especially if pregnant, nursing, or on medication.

• Holy Basil (Ocimum sanctum): Known as Tulsi, it has been used in Ayurvedic medicine to enhance the body's stress response and promote mental clarity.

  - Preparation: Holy Basil can be consumed as tea, in capsules, or as an essential oil for aromatherapy.

- Dosage: For tea, steep 1-2 teaspoons of dried leaves in boiling water for 5-10 minutes. Drink 1-3 cups daily.

- Safety Rating: ♥♥♥♥♡. Generally safe, but pregnant women should avoid due to potential effects on hormone levels.

• Lemon Balm (Melissa officinalis): This herb is known for its calming effects on the nervous system, making it effective in reducing anxiety and promoting relaxation.

- Preparation: Lemon balm can be taken as tea, in capsules, or used in aromatherapy.

- Dosage: For tea, steep 1-2 teaspoons of dried lemon balm in hot water for 10 minutes. Drink up to 4 cups daily.

- Safety Rating: ♥♥♥♥♡. Well-tolerated, but consult a healthcare provider if taking thyroid medication, as it may interact.

Herbs for Improving Sleep

• Valerian Root (Valeriana officinalis): Valerian is widely used for its sedative properties, helping to improve sleep quality and ease insomnia.

- Preparation: Available in capsules, tinctures, or as a tea.

- Dosage: For tea, steep 1 teaspoon of dried root in boiling water for 10 minutes. Drink 30 minutes before bedtime.

- Safety Rating: ♥♥♥♡♡. Avoid long-term use and do not combine with other sedatives.

• Chamomile (Matricaria chamomilla): Renowned for its gentle, soothing effect, chamomile is a popular choice for promoting relaxation and sleep.

- Preparation: Chamomile tea is the most common form, but it can also be taken as capsules or used in aromatherapy.

- Dosage: For tea, steep 2-3 teaspoons of dried chamomile flowers in hot water for 10 minutes. Drink before bedtime.

- Safety Rating: ❤❤❤❤♡. Rare allergic reactions in individuals sensitive to the Asteraceae family.

• Passionflower (Passiflora incarnata): This herb is effective in treating anxiety and insomnia, helping to increase GABA levels in the brain, which promotes relaxation.

- Preparation: Passionflower can be consumed as tea, in capsules, or as a tincture.

- Dosage: For tea, steep 1 teaspoon of dried herb in boiling water for 10 minutes. Drink 1 hour before bedtime.

- Safety Rating: ❤❤❤❤♡. Generally safe, but pregnant and breastfeeding women should avoid.

Incorporating these herbs into your daily routine can offer a natural path to enhanced mental well-being and improved sleep quality. However, it's crucial to consult with a healthcare provider before beginning any herbal regimen, especially if you have existing health conditions or are taking medications.

By understanding the uses, preparations, and safety considerations of these herbs, you can make informed choices about incorporating herbal remedies into your mental health care strategy.

Natural treatments for acne, eczema, and other skin issues.

Skin conditions such as acne, eczema, and psoriasis can be both physically uncomfortable and emotionally distressing. Fortunately, the natural world provides a plethora of herbs known for their soothing, healing, and anti-inflammatory properties, offering relief for these common skin issues. By understanding how to utilize these plants, individuals can explore gentle and effective alternatives to conventional treatments.

Aloe Vera (Aloe barbadensis miller)

Aloe vera is celebrated for its cooling, moisturizing, and healing effects on the skin. It is particularly effective in soothing burns, sunburns, and minor wounds, and its anti-inflammatory properties make it beneficial for acne and eczema.

- Preparation: Apply pure aloe vera gel directly to the affected area. For enhanced effects, the gel can be refrigerated before application.

- Dosage: Apply 2-3 times daily or as needed to soothe irritation.

- Safety Considerations: Topical use of aloe vera gel is generally safe. Ensure the product is free from added colors, fragrances, or alcohol, which can irritate sensitive skin.

Tea Tree Oil (Melaleuca alternifolia)

Tea tree oil is renowned for its potent antimicrobial and anti-inflammatory properties, making it an excellent choice for treating acne. It helps to reduce redness, swelling, and inflammation, and can also prevent and reduce acne scars, leaving the skin smooth and clear.

- Preparation: Dilute tea tree oil with a carrier oil (such as coconut or almond oil) before applying to the skin. A typical dilution ratio is 1-2 drops of tea tree oil per tablespoon of carrier oil.

- Dosage: Apply to the affected area once or twice daily with a cotton swab.

- Safety Considerations: Never apply undiluted tea tree oil directly to the skin as it can cause irritation. Patch test on a small area of skin before full application.

Calendula (Calendula officinalis)

Calendula is known for its anti-inflammatory, antifungal, and antibacterial properties that can help heal wounds, soothe eczema, and relieve diaper rash. It is gentle on the skin and helps in improving skin hydration and firmness.

- Preparation: Use calendula-infused oil or cream on the affected skin areas.

- Dosage: Apply to the skin 2-3 times daily or as needed.

- Safety Considerations: Calendula is generally safe for most people. However, those with allergies to plants in the Asteraceae family should proceed with caution.

Chamomile (Matricaria chamomilla)

Chamomile is not only soothing to the mind but also calming to the skin. Its anti-inflammatory and antioxidant properties make it beneficial for treating skin irritations like eczema, rosacea, and acne.

- Preparation: Apply chamomile tea directly to the skin using a clean cloth or cotton pad, or use skincare products containing chamomile extract.

- Dosage: For direct application, steep 1-2 chamomile tea bags in boiling water for 5 minutes, let cool, and apply to the skin once daily or as needed.

- Safety Considerations: Chamomile is generally safe for topical use. However, individuals with allergies to plants in the Asteraceae family should test a small area first.

Witch Hazel (Hamamelis virginiana)

Witch hazel is widely used for its skin cleansing and toning properties. It can reduce inflammation and soothe sensitive or irritated skin, making it a useful treatment for acne, eczema, and psoriasis.

- Preparation: Apply witch hazel extract with a cotton pad to cleanse and soothe the affected area.

- Dosage: Use 1-2 times daily after washing the face or affected area.

- Safety Considerations: Choose a witch hazel extract that is alcohol-free to avoid drying out the skin.

Incorporating these natural remedies into your skincare routine can offer relief and improvement for various skin conditions. Always conduct a patch test before trying a new treatment, and consult with a healthcare provider if you have severe or persistent skin issues. By leveraging the healing power of herbs, you can nurture your skin back to health gently and effectively.

Women's Health

Herbal approaches to women's health focus on harnessing the natural properties of plants to support menstruation, menopause, and overall reproductive health.

These remedies offer a holistic way to address the unique health challenges women face throughout their lives, from regulating menstrual cycles to easing menopausal symptoms. Understanding how to utilize specific herbs can empower women to manage their health naturally.

Menstrual Health

• Chaste Tree Berry (Vitex agnus-castus): Known for its ability to regulate hormonal imbalances, Chaste Tree Berry is beneficial in easing premenstrual syndrome (PMS) and regulating menstrual cycles.

  - Preparation: Available in capsules or tinctures.

  - Dosage: Follow manufacturer's instructions; typically, 400-500 mg of capsules daily or 1-2 ml of tincture in water, once daily in the morning.

  - Safety Considerations: Generally safe, but consult a healthcare provider before use, especially if using hormonal contraceptives.

• Red Raspberry Leaf (Rubus idaeus): This herb is a uterine tonic that can strengthen and tone the uterine muscles, helping to ease menstrual cramps and improve menstrual regularity.

  - Preparation: Brewed as tea.

  - Dosage: 1-2 teaspoons of dried leaves steeped in boiling water for 10-15 minutes, drunk 1-3 times daily.

  - Safety Considerations: Safe for most individuals, but it's wise to consult a healthcare provider if pregnant.

Menopausal Support

• Black Cohosh (Actaea racemosa): Effective in reducing hot flashes, night sweats, and other menopausal symptoms by acting on estrogen receptors.

  - Preparation: Available in capsules, tinctures, or standardized extracts.

  - Dosage: Follow manufacturer's instructions; typically, 20-40 mg of standardized extract twice daily.

  - Safety Considerations: Short-term use is generally safe; however, it should not be used by individuals with liver disorders and should be discussed with a healthcare provider.

• Dong Quai (Angelica sinensis): Often referred to as "female ginseng," Dong Quai is used to enrich blood, promote circulation, and regulate the menstrual cycle, making it beneficial during menopause for balancing hormones.

  - Preparation: Available in capsules, tinctures, or as part of herbal blends.

  - Dosage: Follow manufacturer's instructions due to varying formulations.

  - Safety Considerations: Should not be used with blood thinners or during pregnancy. Consult a healthcare provider before use.

Reproductive Health

• Maca (Lepidium meyenii): A root known for its ability to enhance fertility and libido by balancing hormone levels and increasing energy.

  - Preparation: Powder added to smoothies, baked goods, or capsules.

- Dosage: 1.5-5 grams of powder daily or as directed for capsules.

- Safety Considerations: Generally safe, but consult a healthcare provider if pregnant or breastfeeding.

• Shatavari (Asparagus racemosus): This adaptogenic herb supports the female reproductive system, aiding in fertility, menstrual regulation, and providing menopausal support by nourishing the body and balancing hormones.

- Preparation: Available in powder or capsules.

- Dosage: 500-1000 mg of capsules daily or 1 teaspoon of powder in warm water twice daily.

- Safety Considerations: Generally safe, but due to its diuretic properties, those with kidney issues should consult a healthcare provider.

Incorporating these herbal remedies into your wellness routine can offer a natural and empowering way to support women's health. It's essential to listen to your body and consult with a healthcare provider before starting any new herbal supplement, especially if you have existing health conditions or are taking medications. By doing so, you can ensure that you are using herbs safely and effectively to support your reproductive health and well-being.

CHAPTER 6: PREPARATION AND USE OF HERBAL REMEDIES

Techniques for Making Herbal Teas and Infusions

Herbal teas and infusions are foundational to practicing herbalism, offering a simple yet effective method for extracting the therapeutic properties of herbs. The process involves steeping dried or fresh herbs in hot water, allowing the water to absorb the flavors and medicinal compounds.

1. Selecting Your Herbs: Choose organic herbs when possible to avoid pesticide exposure. For teas, both dried and fresh herbs can be used, with dried herbs generally having a stronger flavor and potency.

2. Boiling Water: Start with fresh, cold water and bring it to a boil. The temperature of the water is crucial; too hot can destroy delicate compounds, while too cool may not extract the full range of benefits.

3. Proportion and Steeping Time: Use about one teaspoon of dried herbs or two teaspoons of fresh herbs per cup of water. Steep for 5 to 15 minutes, covered, to prevent the escape of aromatic compounds. Longer steeping times result in a stronger tea but may also bring out more bitterness.

4. Straining: Use a fine mesh strainer to separate the herbs from the liquid. Compost the used herbs if possible to minimize waste.

5. Serving: Herbal teas can be enjoyed hot or cold. Sweeteners or lemon might be added for taste, though many prefer to enjoy the pure flavor of the herb.

❤❤❤♡♡ Environmental impact is minimal, especially when using home-grown or locally sourced herbs and composting the remains.

Tinctures and Extracts

Tinctures are concentrated herbal extracts made using alcohol as the solvent. They are valued for their long shelf life and ease of use.

1. Choosing Your Solvent: While alcohol is the most common solvent due to its efficiency in extracting a wide range of compounds and preserving the tincture, glycerin or vinegar can be used as non-alcoholic alternatives.

2. Herb-to-Solvent Ratio: A common ratio is 1:5 (herb weight in grams to solvent volume in milliliters) for dried herbs and 1:2 for fresh herbs. This can vary based on the herb's water content and the desired strength.

3. Maceration: Place the herbs in a clean, dry jar, and cover them with the solvent. Seal the jar tightly and label it with the date and contents. Store the jar in a cool, dark place, shaking it daily for 4 to 6 weeks.

4. Straining: After maceration, strain the mixture through a cheesecloth or fine mesh strainer, squeezing out as much liquid as possible. Transfer the liquid to a clean, dark glass bottle for storage.

5. Usage: Tinctures are typically administered in small doses, often ranging from a few drops to a couple of milliliters, depending on the herb and the individual's needs.

★★☆☆☆ Difficulty level due to the need for precise measurements and patience during the maceration process.

Salves and Balms

Creating salves and balms is a rewarding way to produce topical treatments for skin and muscle issues.

1. Base Ingredients: Start with a base of beeswax and oil. Common choices include coconut oil, olive oil, or almond oil for their skin-nourishing properties. The beeswax thickens the mixture, while the oil carries the medicinal properties of the herbs.

2. Herbal Infusion: Infuse the oil with your chosen herbs either by gently heating the oil and herbs together over a double boiler for 2 to 3

hours or by letting the herbs infuse in the oil at room temperature for 4 to 6 weeks.

3. Melting and Mixing: Once the oil is infused, strain out the herbs. Melt beeswax in a double boiler, then slowly add the infused oil, stirring constantly until fully blended.

4. Pouring and Setting: Pour the mixture into clean tins or jars. Let it cool and solidify before sealing with a lid.

5. Application: Apply the salve or balm directly to the skin as needed for relief from conditions like dry skin, eczema, or muscle pain.

★★★☆☆ Difficulty level, as it requires careful handling of hot ingredients and precise ratios.

Essential Oils

Essential oils are concentrated plant extracts obtained through distillation or mechanical pressing. While not covered in-depth here due to the complexity of their production, their use in aromatherapy and topical applications is widespread.

- Aromatherapy: Essential oils can be diffused into the air to be inhaled or added to baths.

- Topical Use: When diluted with a carrier oil, essential oils can be applied to the skin for various benefits. Always perform a patch test to check for allergic reactions.

❤❤♡♡♡ Safety rating due to the potential for skin irritation or allergic reactions if not properly diluted.

By understanding and applying these preparation techniques, individuals can harness the healing power of herbs in various forms, tailoring their use to personal needs and preferences. Whether seeking to soothe a cough with a warm herbal tea or to ease muscle pain with a homemade salve, the art of herbal remedy preparation is a valuable skill for natural wellness.

Techniques FOR Making Herbal Teas and Infusions: Techniques for herbal beverages.

To craft a nourishing herbal tea or infusion, begin by selecting high-quality, organic herbs. The choice between fresh and dried herbs hinges on personal preference and availability, with dried herbs typically offering a more concentrated flavor.

• Gathering Your Materials: Ensure you have a teapot or a cup, a strainer, and your chosen herbs at hand. For a more potent infusion, a jar with a lid can be used to allow the herbs to steep overnight.

• Water Quality: The foundation of a good herbal tea is water. Use filtered or spring water for the cleanest taste and to avoid any interference with the herb's medicinal properties.

• Heating the Water: Bring your water to just below boiling. For most herbs, water heated to 200-212°F (93-100°C) is ideal. Some delicate herbs, such as green tea leaves, may require cooler water to preserve their subtle flavors and beneficial compounds.

• Herb-to-Water Ratio: A general guideline is to use one teaspoon of dried herbs or two teaspoons of fresh herbs for each cup (8 ounces) of water. Adjust according to taste and the herb's strength.

• Steeping Time: Place the herbs in your teapot or cup and pour the hot water over them. Cover and allow to steep. For a light, delicate flavor, steep for 5-10 minutes. For a stronger infusion, especially with roots or barks, steep for 15 minutes to several hours. An overnight infusion in a jar will extract a maximum amount of nutrients and flavors.

• Straining and Serving: Once the desired steeping time is reached, strain the herbs from the liquid using a fine mesh strainer. Your herbal tea can be enjoyed immediately, served hot, or cooled for a refreshing cold beverage. Personalize your tea with a touch of honey, lemon, or ginger for added flavor.

✓ Remember, the potency of herbs can vary greatly, so start with the recommended amounts and adjust based on personal preference and the specific herb's strength.

♥♥♥♡♡ The environmental impact of making herbal teas and infusions is relatively low, especially when using herbs grown in your garden or sourced from sustainable, organic farms. Composting the spent herbs further minimizes waste and contributes to a cycle of sustainability.

By embracing the simple art of making herbal teas and infusions, you invite the ancient wisdom of herbal healing into your daily routine, connecting with the natural world in a deeply personal and healthful way. Whether seeking relaxation with a cup of chamomile tea before bed or invigoration with a peppermint infusion, the practice of brewing herbal beverages is a versatile and enjoyable aspect of herbalism.

Tinctures and Extracts: How to prepare and use alcohol-based herbal extracts.

Tinctures and extracts are potent, alcohol-based preparations that capture the medicinal properties of herbs in a concentrated form. They are highly valued for their long shelf life and ease of assimilation, making them a staple in herbal medicine cabinets. Here's how to prepare and use them effectively:

Gathering Materials

Before you begin, ensure you have the following items:

- Dried or fresh herbs of your choice

- High-proof alcohol (at least 40% alcohol by volume, such as vodka or brandy)

- A clean, dry glass jar with a tight-fitting lid

- Cheesecloth or a fine mesh strainer

- Amber or blue glass bottles for storage

Preparation Steps

1. Herb Preparation: If using fresh herbs, chop them finely to increase the surface area for extraction. Dried herbs should be lightly crushed or bruised.

2. Filling the Jar: Fill the glass jar about halfway with herbs. This does not need to be precise, but ensure there's enough room left for the alcohol to fully saturate the herbs.

3. Adding Alcohol: Pour the alcohol over the herbs until they are completely submerged. Leave about an inch of space at the top of the jar. The general rule of thumb for the herb-to-alcohol ratio is 1:5 for dried herbs and 1:2 for fresh herbs.

4. Sealing and Labeling: Secure the lid tightly and label the jar with the date and contents. This is crucial for tracking the maceration period and identifying the tincture later.

5. Maceration: Store the jar in a cool, dark place. Shake it daily to encourage extraction. The maceration process should last for 4 to 6 weeks, allowing the alcohol to extract the active constituents from the herbs.

6. Straining: After the maceration period, strain the tincture through cheesecloth or a fine mesh strainer into a clean bowl. Squeeze or press the marc (the leftover herb material) to extract as much liquid as possible.

7. Bottling: Transfer the strained liquid into amber or blue glass bottles. These colored bottles help protect the tincture from light, preserving its potency. If possible, use bottles with dropper caps for easy dosing.

Usage Guidelines

- Dosing: The standard dose for most tinctures is 1-2 ml, taken 2-3 times daily. However, the dose can vary depending on the herb's potency and the individual's sensitivity. Always start with the lower dose to assess tolerance.

- Administration: Tinctures can be taken directly under the tongue for fast absorption into the bloodstream. Alternatively, they can be diluted in a small amount of water or tea.

- Storage: Store tinctures in a cool, dark place. Properly prepared and stored, they can last for several years.

Safety Considerations

- Alcohol Sensitivity: For those with alcohol sensitivities, tinctures can be evaporated in hot water to reduce alcohol content just before use.

- Pregnancy and Breastfeeding: Consult a healthcare provider before using any herbal tinctures during pregnancy or breastfeeding.

- Interactions: Be aware of potential interactions between the herbs in your tincture and any medications you may be taking. Consult with a healthcare professional if unsure.

Tinctures offer a convenient and effective way to utilize the healing power of herbs. By following these steps, you can prepare your own herbal extracts, tailored to your health needs and preferences. Remember, the key to successful tincture making is patience and attention to detail, ensuring you capture the full therapeutic potential of your chosen herbs.

Salves and Balms: How to Creating topical treatments for skin and muscle issues.

Creating salves and balms is a deeply rewarding process that allows you to harness the healing power of herbs in a form that's convenient and directly applicable to the skin. These topical treatments are ideal for addressing a wide range of skin and muscle issues, from dry skin and eczema to sore muscles and inflammation. Here's how to create your own herbal salves and balms:

Preparing the Workspace

1. Clean your workspace thoroughly to prevent contamination.

2. Gather all necessary equipment, including a double boiler, spatulas, measuring cups, and containers for the finished product.

Gathering Materials

- Beeswax, as the base for the salve or balm, provides a protective layer on the skin.

- Carrier oils (such as coconut, olive, or almond oil) to dilute and carry the medicinal properties of the herbs into the skin.

- Dried herbs of choice, depending on the desired effect (e.g., calendula for skin healing, arnica for bruises and soreness).

- Essential oils for added therapeutic benefits and fragrance (optional).

Environmental Impact

Creating your own salves and balms can significantly reduce environmental impact by minimizing packaging waste and allowing for the use of organic, locally sourced ingredients.

Cost Estimate

The initial setup cost may be moderate as you purchase bulk ingredients and equipment. However, homemade salves and balms are generally more cost-effective in the long run compared to store-bought equivalents.

Time Estimate

Expect to spend 2-3 hours preparing and making your salve or balm, including cleanup. The actual cooking time is relatively short, but preparation and cooling can extend the process.

Step-by-Step Instructions

1. Infuse the Carrier Oil: Begin by infusing your carrier oil with the chosen herbs. This can be done through a slow, gentle heat method using a double boiler, where the oil and herbs are heated together for 2-3 hours, or by allowing the herbs to infuse in the oil at room temperature for 4-6 weeks.

2. Strain the Herbs: Once the oil is infused, strain the herbs using a cheesecloth or fine mesh strainer, ensuring all plant material is removed.

3. Melt the Beeswax: In a double boiler, melt the beeswax. Start with a ratio of 1 part beeswax to 4 parts infused oil, adjusting as needed depending on the desired consistency.

4. Combine Oil and Beeswax: Once the beeswax is melted, slowly add the infused oil to the double boiler, stirring constantly until the mixture is fully blended.

5. Add Essential Oils: If using, add a few drops of essential oil to the mixture after removing it from the heat, stirring well to combine.

6. Pour into Containers: Carefully pour the hot mixture into clean, dry containers. Small tins, jars, or even lip balm tubes work well depending on the intended use.

7. Cool and Solidify: Allow the salves or balms to cool completely at room temperature. This may take several hours depending on the size of the containers.

8. Label and Store: Label your containers with the ingredients and date made. Store in a cool, dry place. Most salves and balms will last for 1-2 years if stored properly.

Safety Tips

- Always perform a patch test with a small amount of the finished product to check for any adverse reactions.

- Ensure all containers and tools are sterilized before use to prevent contamination.

Project Variations

- Experiment with different herb and oil combinations to target specific issues. For example, a combination of lavender and chamomile can be soothing for skin irritations, while peppermint and eucalyptus might offer relief for congested chests.

- Consider adding natural colorants or vitamin E oil for additional benefits and preservation.

Additional Considerations

- Be mindful of the melting point of beeswax and the flash points of any essential oils used to ensure safety during the making process.

- Keep detailed notes on your recipes and adjustments for future reference and consistency.

★★★☆☆ Difficulty level due to the need for precision in measurements and understanding the properties of the ingredients. However, with practice, making salves and balms can become an enjoyable and rewarding part of your herbalism practice.

Essential Oils: The benefits and uses of essential oils in aromatherapy and topical applications

Essential oils, the highly concentrated extracts from plants, offer a myriad of benefits and applications that have been utilized for centuries. Their potent properties make them a staple in both aromatherapy and topical applications, providing a natural and effective means to enhance physical and emotional well-being.

Aromatherapy Uses

Aromatherapy involves the inhalation of essential oil vapors to stimulate brain function, impacting mood, mental state, and health. Here are some common ways to use essential oils for aromatherapy:

- Diffusing: Adding a few drops of essential oils to a diffuser can purify the air, promote relaxation, and create a calming atmosphere in any room. For instance, lavender oil is renowned for its ability to reduce stress and improve sleep quality.

- Inhalation: Direct inhalation, such as breathing in the scent from a bottle or a handkerchief dabbed with a few drops of oil, can offer immediate relief from nasal congestion or anxiety. Eucalyptus oil is particularly effective for respiratory issues.

- Baths: Adding essential oils to a warm bath combines the therapeutic effects of water with the benefits of aromatherapy, creating a relaxing and rejuvenating experience. A blend of chamomile and frankincense can soothe the mind and body.

Topical Applications

When applied to the skin, essential oils can offer localized benefits, addressing issues like muscle pain, skin conditions, and wound healing. It's crucial to dilute essential oils with a carrier oil, such as coconut or jojoba oil, to minimize skin sensitivity. Here are some topical uses:

- Massage: Massaging diluted essential oils into the skin can relieve sore muscles, improve circulation, and reduce stress. Peppermint oil, for example, is excellent for easing tension headaches and muscle aches.

- Skincare: Essential oils can be added to lotions or creams to address skin concerns. Tea tree oil, with its antimicrobial properties, is effective against acne, while rosehip oil can help reduce signs of aging.

- Wound Care: Some essential oils can support the healing of minor cuts and burns. Lavender oil, known for its antimicrobial and soothing properties, can be applied to a wound to promote healing and reduce scarring.

Safety and Dilution

- Patch Test: Always perform a patch test before using a new essential oil topically to ensure there's no allergic reaction.

- Dilution: Essential oils should be diluted with a carrier oil to prevent irritation. A general guideline is to use a 2% dilution, which is about 12 drops of essential oil per ounce of carrier oil.

- Sensitive Areas: Avoid applying essential oils near sensitive areas, such as the eyes, ears, and mucous membranes.

Environmental and Ethical Considerations

Choosing sustainably sourced and organic essential oils not only supports the environment but also ensures the purity and efficacy of the oils. Ethical sourcing practices respect the labor and traditions of indigenous communities and contribute to the conservation of plant species.

Essential oils bridge the gap between traditional herbal practices and modern wellness, offering a versatile and effective approach to health. Whether used in aromatherapy or applied topically, these potent extracts can significantly enhance the quality of life, providing a natural complement to conventional health care practices.

CHAPTER 7: SAFETY AND ETHICS IN HERBALISM

Dosage and Toxicity

Understanding the correct dosage of herbal remedies is crucial for their safe and effective use. Herbs, like any form of medicine, can have adverse effects if used improperly. The therapeutic window—the range between effectiveness and toxicity—can vary widely among different herbs and individuals. Factors such as age, weight, health condition, and concurrent use of other medications must be considered when determining dosage.

• Start Low, Go Slow: Begin with the lowest recommended dose and gradually increase as needed. This approach helps identify the minimum effective dose and reduces the risk of adverse effects.

• Consult Reliable Sources: Use dosage guidelines from reputable sources or consult with a healthcare professional experienced in herbal medicine.

• Be Aware of Potent Herbs: Some herbs, such as foxglove (Digitalis purpurea) and wormwood (Artemisia absinthium), contain powerful compounds that can be toxic in small amounts. Always exercise caution and seek professional guidance when using potent herbs.

Interactions with Pharmaceuticals

Herbs can interact with prescription and over-the-counter medications, sometimes with dangerous consequences. These interactions can enhance or diminish the effect of medications, leading to under-treatment or toxic side effects.

• Consult Healthcare Providers: Before adding an herbal remedy to your regimen, discuss it with a healthcare provider, especially if you are taking medications for chronic conditions.

• Use a Comprehensive Approach: Inform all your healthcare providers about every remedy and medication you are taking to ensure a holistic understanding of your treatment plan.

• Monitor for Side Effects: Be vigilant for any new symptoms or changes in health status and report them to a healthcare provider promptly.

Ethical Harvesting

Sustainable and ethical harvesting practices are essential to protect plant species from overharvesting and to ensure that herbal remedies are available for future generations. Ethical harvesting also respects the rights and traditions of indigenous peoples and local communities who have used these plants for centuries.

• Support Sustainable Sources: Purchase herbs from suppliers who prioritize sustainability and ethical sourcing practices.

• Wildcrafting with Respect: If you harvest herbs from the wild, take only what you need, leave plenty for regeneration, and be mindful not to damage the plant's habitat.

• Cultivate Your Own: Whenever possible, grow your own herbs. This not only ensures a sustainable supply but also deepens your connection to the plants you use for healing.

Safety and Ethics in Herbalism

The practice of herbalism carries with it a responsibility to both the individual and the environment. By adhering to guidelines on dosage and toxicity, being mindful of interactions with pharmaceuticals, and committing to ethical harvesting practices, herbalists can ensure that their practice is safe, effective, and sustainable. Remember, the goal of herbalism is to support health and well-being, both of which are best served when safety and ethics guide the way.

Dosage and Toxicity: Understanding safe dosages and potential toxicities of certain herbs.

Navigating the realm of herbal remedies requires a nuanced understanding of dosage and toxicity. Herbs, while natural, are not without their risks, and their therapeutic efficacy is deeply intertwined with the quantities in which they are consumed. The adage "the dose makes the poison" holds true in herbalism, underscoring the importance of respecting the potency of plants.

• Individual Sensitivities and Conditions: The optimal dosage of an herb can vary significantly among individuals, influenced by factors such as age, body weight, metabolic rate, and overall health. For instance, children and the elderly often require lower doses due to their different metabolic capacities. Similarly, individuals with certain health conditions or those who are pregnant may need to adjust dosages or avoid certain herbs altogether.

• Understanding Standard Dosages: Most herbs come with recommended dosages based on traditional use and contemporary research. These guidelines serve as a starting point, but it's crucial to adjust based on personal tolerance and response. For teas, a common recommendation might be 1-2 teaspoons of dried herb per cup of water, steeped for 10-15 minutes. Tinctures, being more concentrated, typically suggest starting with 1-2 milliliters, 2-3 times a day. However, these are merely guidelines, not one-size-fits-all prescriptions.

• Recognizing Signs of Toxicity: Overconsumption of certain herbs can lead to adverse effects, ranging from mild (e.g., gastrointestinal discomfort, headaches) to severe (e.g., liver damage, neurological symptoms). It's vital to be aware of the specific signs of toxicity associated with each herb and to cease consumption immediately if adverse reactions occur. For example, excessive use of licorice root can lead to hypertension and potassium depletion, while too much St. John's Wort may cause photosensitivity and interact with conventional medications.

• Interactions with Pharmaceuticals: Many herbs can interact with prescription medications, either enhancing their effects (leading to potential overdose) or inhibiting them (reducing their therapeutic benefit). Such interactions can also increase the risk of side effects. Before incorporating an herbal remedy into your regimen, consult with a healthcare provider, especially if you are taking medications for chronic conditions.

• Long-Term Use Considerations: While some herbs can be safely consumed over long periods, others are best used in shorter cycles to prevent potential toxicity or diminishing returns. Adaptogens, for example, are often taken in cycles to maintain their efficacy and minimize the risk of side effects.

66

• Special Populations: Pregnant and breastfeeding women, children, and those with pre-existing health conditions should exercise extra caution with herbal remedies. Many herbs are contraindicated in pregnancy and lactation due to their potential to affect hormonal balance or because their safety profiles are not well-established.

Incorporating herbs into one's wellness routine should be done with mindfulness and respect for the plants' power. Starting with lower doses and gradually adjusting based on personal response can help mitigate risks. Additionally, staying informed about the latest research and consulting with healthcare professionals experienced in herbal medicine are prudent steps to ensure safe and effective use. By approaching herbalism with a balanced perspective on dosage and toxicity, individuals can harness the healing potential of plants while minimizing the risk of adverse effects.

Interactions with Pharmaceuticals

Herbal remedies have been used for centuries to treat a myriad of ailments, offering natural alternatives to conventional medicines. However, as the use of herbal supplements becomes increasingly popular, it's crucial to understand how they can interact with pharmaceutical medications. These interactions can either diminish the effectiveness of your medication, enhance its effects to a dangerous level, or even introduce new side effects.

• Mechanisms of Interaction: Herbal remedies can interact with pharmaceuticals through various mechanisms. Some herbs may increase the metabolism of medications, leading to decreased drug levels and effectiveness. Conversely, certain herbs can inhibit the metabolism of drugs, increasing their levels and potential toxicity. For example, St. John's Wort is known to induce the cytochrome P450 enzyme system, potentially reducing the effectiveness of medications metabolized by these enzymes, such as some antidepressants, birth control pills, and anticoagulants.

• Risks of Bleeding: Herbs like Ginkgo biloba, garlic, and high doses of fish oil have anticoagulant properties, which can increase the risk of bleeding when taken with blood-thinning medications like warfarin or aspirin.

• Blood Pressure Variations: Herbal supplements such as licorice can elevate blood pressure and may interfere with antihypertensive drugs, reducing their efficacy. Conversely, herbs like hawthorn can potentiate the effects of blood pressure medications, leading to hypotension.

• Blood Sugar Control: For individuals managing diabetes with medication, it's important to be cautious with herbs like fenugreek, cinnamon, and bitter melon, which can lower blood sugar levels. These herbs may enhance the effects of diabetes medications, potentially leading to hypoglycemia.

• Central Nervous System Effects: Herbs such as valerian root and kava can enhance the sedative effects of CNS depressants, including benzodiazepines and some types of antidepressants, leading to increased drowsiness and decreased motor coordination.

• Consulting Healthcare Providers: Always inform your healthcare provider about any herbal supplements you are taking or considering. This is especially important if you are on medications for chronic conditions such as heart disease, diabetes, or depression. A healthcare provider can offer guidance on safe herbal use and monitor for potential interactions.

• Being Informed: Educate yourself about the herbal remedies you are interested in. Reliable sources include peer-reviewed journals, professional healthcare providers, and reputable health websites. Knowledge about the specific actions of an herb, its potential side effects, and interactions with medications can help you make informed decisions about your health.

• Monitoring for Side Effects: If you're taking both herbal remedies and pharmaceutical medications, be vigilant for any new or unusual symptoms. Side effects that may seem minor, such as fatigue or gastrointestinal disturbances, could be early indicators of an interaction. Report any adverse effects to your healthcare provider promptly. Incorporating herbal remedies into your healthcare regimen can offer benefits, but it's essential to do so with awareness and caution, especially when pharmaceutical medications are involved. By understanding the potential for interactions, consulting with healthcare professionals, and staying informed, you can safely navigate the use of herbal remedies alongside modern medications.

Ethical Harvesting

Ethical harvesting encompasses a set of practices that ensure the sustainability of plant species and respect for the lands and cultures from which these plants are derived. As herbalists and enthusiasts, adopting ethical harvesting practices is not only a matter of environmental responsibility but also a gesture of respect towards the intricate web of life that includes plants, humans, and the ecosystem at large. Here are key considerations and steps to ensure ethical harvesting:

• Knowledge of the Plant Species: Before harvesting any plant, it's crucial to have a thorough understanding of its growth cycle, abundance, and ecological role. This knowledge helps in determining the right time to harvest, ensuring that the plant can regenerate and continue to thrive in its habitat.

• Permission and Legal Considerations: Always seek permission before harvesting plants, especially if you are on private land or in protected areas. Familiarize yourself with local, state, and federal regulations regarding wild plant harvesting to ensure compliance with conservation laws.

• Sustainable Harvesting Techniques: Practice sustainable harvesting by taking only what you need and leaving enough plant material so the population can regenerate. For example, when harvesting leaves or flowers, take only a small portion from each plant, leaving the rest to continue its growth cycle.

• Respecting Traditional Knowledge: Many plants have been used medicinally for centuries by indigenous and local communities. It's important to acknowledge and respect this traditional knowledge, avoiding the commercial exploitation of plants that are sacred or crucial to these communities. Engage with and learn from these communities, ensuring that your harvesting practices do not deplete resources they depend on.

• Cultivation as an Alternative: Whenever possible, cultivate your own medicinal plants. This not only reduces pressure on wild plant populations but also gives you control over the growing conditions, ensuring that your herbs are free from pesticides and other contaminants.

• Leave No Trace: When harvesting in the wild, practice the principle of "leave no trace." This means not only taking care not to damage the plant and its surroundings but also ensuring that you do not leave any waste behind.

• Document and Share Knowledge: Keep a record of your harvesting practices, including the locations, times of year, and methods used. Sharing this information with fellow herbalists and conservationists can help spread awareness of ethical practices and encourage a community-wide commitment to sustainability.

By adhering to these ethical harvesting practices, herbalists can contribute to the preservation of plant species and their habitats, ensuring that these natural resources remain abundant for future generations. Moreover, respecting traditional knowledge and engaging with indigenous and local communities in a manner that honors their cultural heritage and expertise enriches the practice of herbalism, making it a more inclusive and holistic discipline.

CHAPTER 8: HERBALISM IN DIFFERENT CULTURES

Herbalism, a practice as ancient as humanity itself, has flourished in diverse cultures around the globe, each developing its unique traditions and approaches to healing with plants. This rich tapestry of global herbal practices offers a fascinating glimpse into how different societies have harnessed the power of the natural world for health and healing.

Traditional Chinese Medicine (TCM)

In China, herbalism is a cornerstone of Traditional Chinese Medicine, a comprehensive health system that views the body as a balance of opposing forces: Yin and Yang. TCM practitioners use an extensive pharmacopeia of herbs to restore harmony and treat illness. Key concepts include:

- Qi (vital energy): Herbal remedies are often prescribed to balance Qi, which is believed to flow through pathways in the body.

- Five Elements Theory: This links the body's health to natural elements (wood, fire, earth, metal, and water), influencing the choice of herbs.

- Herbal Formulas: Unlike Western herbalism, which may use single herbs, TCM combines multiple herbs in precise ratios to create complex formulas tailored to the individual's condition.

Ayurveda

Originating in India over 3,000 years ago, Ayurveda is another holistic healing system that incorporates herbalism. It emphasizes the balance among three elemental energies or doshas (Vata, Pitta, and Kapha). Ayurvedic herbalism is characterized by:

- Personalization: Herbs and treatments are selected based on the individual's dominant dosha and the specific imbalances they are experiencing.

- Rasayanas: These are herbal formulations believed to promote longevity and rejuvenation.

- Panchakarma: A cleansing process that may include herbal oil massages, steam baths, and other methods to detoxify the body.

Indigenous Knowledge

Across the Americas, Africa, Australia, and other regions, indigenous peoples have developed their own rich herbal traditions, deeply intertwined with their cultural beliefs and practices. Common themes include:

- Spiritual Aspect: Many indigenous cultures view illness as a disharmony between the individual and their environment or spiritual world, with herbs often used in ritual contexts.

- Local Flora: Indigenous herbalism makes extensive use of local plants, many of which are unique to their specific regions and have been passed down through generations.

- Holistic Approach: Like TCM and Ayurveda, indigenous herbal practices often consider the physical, emotional, and spiritual well-being of the person.

Integration and Challenges

As herbalism continues to gain popularity worldwide, integrating these diverse traditions into modern healthcare poses both opportunities and challenges. Issues of intellectual property, sustainability, and ensuring the quality and safety of herbal products are paramount. Moreover, respecting the cultural origins and knowledge of indigenous and traditional practices is crucial in this global exchange.

The Future of Global Herbal Traditions

The future of herbalism lies in a respectful, informed integration of these diverse cultural practices, contributing to a more holistic and personalized approach to health and wellness. As research into herbal medicine advances, it is essential to maintain a dialogue between traditional knowledge and scientific inquiry, ensuring that the benefits of herbalism are accessible to all, while preserving the wisdom of the past.

In exploring the herbal traditions of different cultures, we not only broaden our understanding of herbalism but also gain insight into the universal human quest for health and balance with nature.

Traditional Chinese Medicine: The role of herbs in TCM.

Traditional Chinese Medicine (TCM) stands as a testament to the enduring power of herbal remedies, woven deeply into the fabric of healthcare for thousands of years. At the heart of TCM lies the profound belief in the interconnectedness of the human body with the natural world, a concept that guides the use of herbs to restore balance and health. The role of herbs in TCM is multifaceted, embodying principles of balance, harmony, and energy flow that are essential for understanding this ancient practice.

Herbs in TCM are not merely seen as substances with biochemical effects but as entities possessing unique energies and properties that can influence the Qi (vital energy), Yin and Yang (the fundamental dual forces of nature), and the Five Elements (wood, fire, earth, metal, and water) within the body. This holistic approach ensures that herbal treatments are tailored to the individual's specific imbalances, rather than adopting a one-size-fits-all methodology.

The practice of combining herbs into formulas is a distinctive characteristic of TCM. These formulas, some of which have been preserved through centuries, are complex mixtures of herbs that work synergistically to address not just symptoms but the root cause of illness. The art of formula preparation is highly sophisticated, with each herb playing a specific role as the principal, assistant, or messenger ingredient, thereby enhancing the formula's effectiveness and minimizing potential side effects.

Key concepts integral to the role of herbs in TCM include:

• Qi Enhancing: Many herbs are selected for their ability to enhance Qi, thereby supporting the body's vital energy and promoting overall well-being. Ginseng, for example, is renowned for its Qi-boosting properties.

• Yin and Yang Balancing: Herbs like Yin Yang Huo (Horny Goat Weed) are used to balance the dynamic interplay of Yin and Yang within the body, essential for maintaining health.

• Five Elements Theory: This theory, which correlates specific organs and functions to natural elements, guides the selection of herbs. For instance, herbs associated with the water element may be used to support kidney health.

• Meridian Targeting: TCM posits that the body is crisscrossed by meridians, or energy pathways, each linked to specific organs. Herbs are chosen for their ability to target and unblock these meridians, facilitating the smooth flow of Qi.

Understanding the role of herbs in TCM requires an appreciation of these underlying principles, which emphasize harmony and balance. It's a system where diagnosis and treatment are deeply personalized, reflecting the unique conditions and needs of each individual. This personalized approach, combined with a rich pharmacopeia of herbs, enables TCM practitioners to treat a wide array of health issues, from chronic diseases to acute conditions, with remarkable nuance and depth.

In embracing the wisdom of TCM, one gains insight into a holistic approach to health that has stood the test of time, offering natural solutions that complement and enhance well-being. The role of herbs in TCM is not just about treating illness; it's about nurturing life's essence, promoting longevity, and harmonizing the body with the natural world.

Ayurveda: Herbal practices in Indian medicine.

Ayurveda, a traditional system of medicine from India, has a rich history that dates back over 3,000 years. It is based on the principle that health and wellness depend on a delicate balance between the mind, body, and spirit. Central to Ayurvedic medicine is the concept of the doshas, three energies that govern physiological activity. These doshas are Vata (space and air), Pitta (fire and water), and Kapha (water and earth), and each individual has a unique combination of these doshas, defining their constitution and health.

Herbalism plays a pivotal role in Ayurveda, with a vast array of plants used not only for their physical healing properties but also for their spiritual and psychological benefits. The use of herbs is tailored to the individual's dosha balance, aiming to detoxify the body, restore balance, and build immunity. Here are some key aspects of Ayurvedic herbal practices:

74

• Personalized Herbal Treatment: Unlike the one-size-fits-all approach, Ayurveda emphasizes personalized herbal remedies. Practitioners carefully select herbs that will balance the specific dosha imbalances of an individual, considering factors such as age, health status, season, and digestive capacity.

• Rasayanas for Rejuvenation: Rasayanas are special herbal formulations used in Ayurveda to rejuvenate the body and mind, enhance longevity, and prevent disease. These formulations often include herbs such as Ashwagandha, Amalaki, and Brahmi, known for their nourishing and revitalizing properties.

• Detoxification and Panchakarma: Ayurveda uses herbal preparations in its detoxification process known as Panchakarma. This intensive cleansing program is designed to eliminate toxins from the body, using herbal oils and substances for massages, enemas, and nasal administrations.

• Herbal Formulations: Ayurvedic medicine commonly uses complex herbal formulations that may include dozens of different herbs. These formulations are designed to work synergistically, enhancing the efficacy of the treatment and reducing potential side effects.

• Diet and Herbal Integration: Ayurveda also integrates herbs into daily diet and lifestyle, recognizing that food itself is medicine. Dietary recommendations are made based on the individual's dominant dosha and may include specific herbs and spices to aid digestion and overall health.

Some commonly used Ayurvedic herbs and their benefits include:

- Turmeric (Curcuma longa): Known for its anti-inflammatory and antioxidant properties, turmeric is used to support joint health, digestion, and skin health.

- Ashwagandha (Withania somnifera): This adaptogen is used to help the body resist stressors, promoting energy, vitality, and overall well-being.

- Triphala: A combination of three fruits, Triphala is a gentle laxative that also supports digestion and detoxification.

- Brahmi (Bacopa monnieri): Brahmi is revered for its mind-enhancing properties, improving memory, concentration, and calming the nervous system.

Incorporating Ayurvedic herbal practices into daily life can offer a holistic approach to health, emphasizing prevention, balance, and the natural healing power of plants. As with any medicinal practice, it's important to consult with a qualified practitioner to ensure the safe and effective use of Ayurvedic herbs, especially when integrating them with other treatments or medications. Ayurveda's holistic approach, with its deep respect for the individual's unique constitution, offers a timeless wisdom that can complement modern healthcare practices, providing a natural pathway to vitality and wellness.

Indigenous Knowledge

Indigenous cultures across the Americas have long harnessed the power of the Earth's flora for healing, spiritual practices, and maintaining balance within the body and with the natural world. The rich herbal traditions of Native American and other indigenous peoples offer a window into a holistic approach to health care that is deeply rooted in the understanding of local ecosystems and the medicinal properties of plants.

Native American herbalism, in particular, is characterized by a profound respect for nature and the belief that every plant has a spirit and purpose. This knowledge, passed down through generations, encompasses not just the physical aspects of healing but also the spiritual, recognizing that health is a balance of mind, body, and spirit. Here are some key aspects of indigenous herbal practices:

• Local Flora Utilization: Indigenous herbalists utilize plants that grow in their immediate environment, reflecting a deep understanding of regional biodiversity. For example, the use of sage for cleansing rituals and echinacea for immune support are well-documented practices among Native American tribes.

• Holistic Healing: The approach to healing is comprehensive, addressing not just physical symptoms but also spiritual and emotional well-being. This might involve the use of herbal remedies in conjunction with rituals, ceremonies, and storytelling to support the healing process.

• Spiritual Connection: Many indigenous traditions hold that before harvesting a plant for medicinal use, one should offer a prayer or token of gratitude. This practice underscores the deep spiritual relationship between healers and the natural world.

• Community and Oral Traditions: Knowledge about medicinal plants and their uses is often shared through oral traditions, passed down from elders to younger generations within a community. This ensures the preservation of cultural identity and knowledge, even in the face of modernization and globalization.

• Integration with Other Healing Practices: Indigenous herbalism is often part of a larger system of healing that includes physical therapies (such as massage and sweat lodges), dietary guidelines, and community healing practices.

Some commonly used plants in indigenous herbalism include:

- White Willow Bark: Used for pain relief and inflammation, similar to the way aspirin is used in Western medicine.

- Cedar: Employed in cleansing rituals and also as a tea for respiratory health.

- Sweetgrass: Burned for its sweet, calming fragrance during ceremonies and believed to attract positive energies.

- Yarrow: Applied topically for wounds and infections or taken internally to aid digestion.

Indigenous herbal practices are a testament to the deep connection between human health and the natural world. They remind us of the importance of respecting and preserving traditional knowledge and biodiversity for future generations. As interest in herbalism grows, it's crucial to approach indigenous practices with respect, seeking permission and guidance from those who hold this knowledge. Engaging with these traditions offers not only insights into effective natural remedies but also a broader perspective on health and wellness that can enrich our modern lives.

CHAPTER 9: FUTURE OF HERBALISM AND NATURAL REMEDIES

The future of herbalism and natural remedies is poised at an exciting crossroads, blending ancient wisdom with cutting-edge science to forge new paths in healthcare. As we look ahead, several key trends and innovations are shaping the way we understand and utilize plant-based medicine. These developments promise to expand the role of herbalism in modern healthcare, making natural remedies more accessible, effective, and integrated into our daily lives.

Integration with Modern Medicine

The integration of herbalism into modern healthcare systems is gaining momentum, driven by a growing body of scientific research that validates the efficacy of many traditional remedies. Hospitals and clinics are increasingly offering complementary and alternative medicine (CAM) services, including herbal consultations, as part of their patient care. This trend is supported by:

- Collaborative Research: Partnerships between herbalists, universities, and pharmaceutical companies are leading to rigorous studies on the safety and effectiveness of herbal remedies.

- Educational Programs: Medical schools are beginning to incorporate courses on herbalism and CAM, equipping new generations of healthcare professionals with a broader understanding of natural therapies.

- Regulatory Frameworks: Governments are developing clearer regulations for herbal products, ensuring they meet standards for quality, safety, and efficacy.

Research and Innovation

The scientific exploration of plants is uncovering new compounds and therapeutic possibilities, pushing the boundaries of how we can harness nature's pharmacy. Key areas of innovation include:

- Phytochemistry: Advanced techniques in phytochemical analysis are identifying active compounds in plants, some of which may lead to the development of new drugs.

- Genetic Engineering: Biotechnology is being used to enhance the medicinal properties of plants, making them more potent or easier to grow.

- Delivery Systems: Innovations in how herbal remedies are administered, such as nanoparticle delivery systems, are improving their bioavailability and effectiveness.

Education and Advocacy

As interest in herbalism grows, so does the need for accurate information and advocacy for its safe and informed use. Efforts in this area include:

- Public Education: Workshops, online courses, and publications are making knowledge about herbalism more accessible to the public.

- Professional Development: Continuing education opportunities for healthcare professionals in herbalism are expanding, fostering a more integrated approach to patient care.

- Policy Advocacy: Herbalists and organizations are advocating for policies that support the sustainable use of medicinal plants and protect traditional knowledge.

The Role of Herbalism in Animal Care

The use of herbal remedies is extending beyond human healthcare to include veterinary practices. Pet owners and farmers are turning to natural remedies to enhance the health and well-being of animals. This trend is supported by:

- Veterinary Herbal Medicine: More veterinarians are incorporating herbal remedies into their practices, offering natural options for pet owners.

- Livestock Health: Herbal supplements are being used to promote the health of livestock, reducing the reliance on antibiotics and supporting sustainable farming practices.

Herbalism and Environmental Health

The future of herbalism is deeply intertwined with the health of our planet. Sustainable practices in the cultivation and harvesting of medicinal plants are critical to ensuring the longevity of herbalism. This includes:

- Conservation Efforts: Protecting wild plant populations and their habitats is essential to preserve biodiversity and the availability of medicinal plants.

- Sustainable Farming: Organic and biodynamic farming practices for medicinal plants are reducing environmental impact and ensuring the purity of herbal remedies.

Advanced Herbal Preparation Techniques

Innovation in herbal preparation techniques is enhancing the potency and purity of natural remedies. Techniques such as fermentation and advanced extraction methods are creating more powerful and targeted herbal products. These advancements include:

- Fermentation: This ancient technique is being revisited to enhance the bioavailability and efficacy of herbal remedies.

- Advanced Extraction: Supercritical CO_2 extraction and other modern methods are producing highly concentrated extracts, offering more potent therapeutic benefits.

The Psychological Effects of Herbalism

The holistic nature of herbalism addresses not only physical health but also mental and emotional well-being. The future of herbalism includes a greater focus on the psychological effects of plant interaction, recognizing the benefits of herbal remedies in supporting mental health and emotional balance.

As we move forward, the future of herbalism and natural remedies is bright, marked by a harmonious blend of tradition and innovation. By embracing the wisdom of the past and the scientific advancements of the present, we can unlock the full potential of herbal medicine to nurture health and well-being in our modern world.

Integration with Modern Medicine: How herbalism is being integrated into modern healthcare.

The integration of herbalism into modern healthcare represents a significant shift towards a more holistic approach to medicine, blending ancient wisdom with contemporary medical practices. This convergence is evident in various aspects of healthcare, from clinical settings to research laboratories, and reflects a growing recognition of the value that herbal medicine can offer in promoting health and wellness.

One of the most visible signs of this integration is the incorporation of herbal remedies into conventional medical treatments. Many healthcare providers now recognize the benefits of combining herbal treatments with traditional medicine to enhance patient care. This approach is particularly prevalent in the management of chronic conditions, where herbal remedies can complement pharmacological treatments to improve outcomes and reduce side effects.

In addition to direct patient care, the integration of herbalism and modern medicine is also advancing through research. Scientific studies on herbal medicine have increased, with researchers exploring the efficacy, safety, and mechanisms of action of various herbs. This research is not only validating the traditional uses of many plants but also uncovering new therapeutic potentials. Collaborations between herbalists, pharmacologists, and biologists are leading to a deeper understanding of how plant compounds interact with human biology, paving the way for the development of novel treatments.

Educational institutions are also playing a crucial role in bridging the gap between herbalism and modern medicine. Medical schools and universities are increasingly offering courses and programs in herbal medicine and complementary therapies, equipping future healthcare professionals with a broader range of tools to support patient health. This education extends beyond the classroom, with professional development workshops and continuing education courses available for practicing clinicians.

Regulatory bodies have responded to the growing integration of herbalism into healthcare by establishing guidelines and standards for herbal products. These regulations ensure that herbal remedies meet quality, safety, and efficacy standards comparable to those of conventional medicines. As a result, patients and healthcare providers can have greater confidence in the herbal treatments used alongside or as part of conventional medical care.

The integration of herbalism into modern healthcare is also evident in the growing number of hospitals and clinics offering integrative medicine services. These services combine the best of conventional and herbal medicine to provide comprehensive care that addresses the physical, emotional, and spiritual aspects of health. Integrative medicine centers often include herbalists on their teams, working alongside doctors, nurses, and other healthcare professionals to create personalized treatment plans for patients.

This blending of herbalism and modern medicine represents a promising development in healthcare, offering a more nuanced and holistic approach to treating illness and promoting wellness. By drawing on the strengths of both traditional and contemporary medical practices, this integration holds the potential to improve patient outcomes, enhance the quality of care, and contribute to the evolution of a more sustainable and patient-centered healthcare system.

Research and Innovation: Current research on herbal medicine and potential future discoveries.

The realm of herbal medicine is currently experiencing an unprecedented surge in research and innovation, with scientists, herbalists, and healthcare professionals working together to unlock the full potential of plants in treating and preventing disease. This collaborative effort is not only validating the traditional uses of herbs but also leading to groundbreaking discoveries that could shape the future of healthcare.

One of the most exciting areas of current research involves the phytochemical analysis of medicinal plants. Advanced technologies such as mass spectrometry and nuclear magnetic resonance spectroscopy are allowing researchers to identify and isolate active compounds in herbs with greater precision than ever before. This meticulous work is the foundation for developing new pharmaceuticals derived from plants, offering hope for treatments that are more effective and have fewer side effects than conventional drugs.

Biotechnology plays a pivotal role in the innovation of herbal medicine, particularly through the genetic modification of plants to enhance their medicinal properties. Scientists are experimenting with ways to increase the concentrations of active compounds in herbs, making them more potent and efficient. Additionally, biotechnology is being used to cultivate rare or endangered medicinal plants in laboratory settings, ensuring their preservation and sustainable use.

Another promising avenue of research is the exploration of novel delivery systems for herbal medicine. Innovations such as nanoparticle carriers and transdermal patches are being developed to improve the bioavailability and efficacy of herbal compounds. These advanced delivery systems could revolutionize the way herbal remedies are administered, making them more convenient and effective for patients.

The exploration of synergistic effects between different herbs and between herbs and conventional medications is also a key focus of current research. Understanding how different compounds interact can lead to the development of more effective herbal formulations and integrated treatment plans that leverage the best of both traditional and modern medicine.

Looking to the future, one of the most anticipated areas of discovery is the potential for herbal medicine to address global health challenges such as antibiotic resistance, chronic diseases, and mental health conditions. With an increasing number of studies supporting the efficacy of herbal treatments, there is hope that herbs could provide viable alternatives or complements to conventional treatments, offering solutions that are both sustainable and accessible.

Furthermore, the growing interest in personalized medicine aligns perfectly with the principles of herbalism, which has always emphasized the importance of tailoring treatments to the individual. Future innovations may include the development of herbal formulations customized to an individual's genetic makeup, lifestyle, and health conditions, maximizing therapeutic benefits and minimizing risks.

Education and Advocacy: How to promote and educate others about the benefits and uses of herbal remedies.

Promoting and educating others about the benefits and uses of herbal remedies is a vital step towards integrating these ancient practices into modern health and wellness routines. The resurgence of interest in herbalism presents an opportunity to share knowledge, dispel myths, and advocate for the safe and effective use of plants for healing. Here are strategies and approaches to effectively educate and advocate for herbal remedies:

1. Leverage Social Media and Online Platforms: Utilize the power of social media, blogs, and online forums to share information, research findings, and personal success stories with herbal remedies. Creating engaging content such as how-to videos, infographics, and live Q&A sessions can help demystify herbalism for the general public.

2. Host Workshops and Seminars: Organize educational events in your community or online to teach people about the basics of herbalism, including plant identification, preparation of remedies, and safety considerations. Hands-on workshops where participants can make their own herbal teas or salves can be particularly engaging.

3. Publish Articles and Books: Writing articles for health and wellness magazines or publishing a book on herbal remedies can reach a wide audience. Focus on topics that resonate with contemporary health concerns, such as stress management, immune support, or natural beauty, and provide evidence-based information to support your claims.

4. Collaborate with Healthcare Professionals: Build relationships with doctors, nurses, and other healthcare providers to share information about the benefits and science behind herbal remedies. Offering to conduct educational sessions for medical staff can help integrate herbalism into more conventional healthcare settings.

5. Advocate for Quality and Safety Standards: Engage in advocacy efforts to support the regulation and quality control of herbal products. This can involve working with policymakers, attending public hearings, or participating in campaigns to ensure that herbal remedies available to consumers are safe and effective.

6. Support Herbal Education in Schools: Advocate for the inclusion of herbalism and plant science in school curriculums. Educating children about the importance of plants and their medicinal properties can

foster a lifelong appreciation for natural remedies and environmental stewardship.

7. Create a Community Herbal Garden: Encourage your community to start a herbal garden as a hands-on educational tool. This not only provides a tangible way to learn about growing and using medicinal plants but also strengthens community bonds and promotes sustainability.

8. Offer Mentorship and Internships: If you are an experienced herbalist, consider mentoring aspiring herbalists or offering internships at your practice. This one-on-one guidance is invaluable for practical learning and can help perpetuate the tradition of herbal healing.

9. Participate in Health Fairs and Community Events: Set up a booth at local health fairs, farmers' markets, and community events to offer information, free samples, and demonstrations on using herbal remedies. Personal interactions can be a powerful way to educate and inspire curiosity about herbalism.

10. Utilize Public Speaking Opportunities: Seek opportunities to speak at conferences, local clubs, and educational institutions about the role of herbal remedies in health and wellness. Tailoring your message to the interests and concerns of your audience can make your presentation more impactful.

By adopting these strategies, herbalists and enthusiasts can play a crucial role in educating the public about the benefits of herbal remedies, advocating for their safe use, and ensuring that the ancient art of herbal healing continues to thrive in the modern world.

CHAPTER 10: THE ROLE OF HERBALISM IN ANIMAL CARE

The integration of herbalism into animal care represents a harmonious blend of traditional knowledge and modern veterinary practices, offering a natural and holistic approach to maintaining the health and well-being of animals. This chapter delves into the practical applications of herbal remedies in veterinary medicine, covering both domestic pets and livestock. It explores the benefits, safety considerations, and preparation methods of herbal treatments, providing a comprehensive guide for pet owners and farmers interested in incorporating herbalism into their animal care routines.

Veterinary Herbal Medicine

Veterinary herbal medicine involves the use of plant-based remedies to prevent and treat a wide range of health conditions in animals. This practice is grounded in the understanding that, just like humans, animals can benefit from the healing properties of plants. Herbal remedies are used to support the immune system, improve digestion, reduce inflammation, and promote overall health and vitality in animals. Key aspects include:

- Herb Selection: Choosing the right herbs is crucial. Commonly used herbs in animal care include chamomile for its calming effects, ginger for digestive health, and turmeric for its anti-inflammatory properties.

- Dosage and Administration: The appropriate dosage varies depending on the animal's size, age, and health condition. Herbal remedies can be administered orally, topically, or added to the animal's food.

- Safety and Efficacy: While many herbs are safe for animals, it's important to consult with a veterinary herbalist to ensure the chosen herbs will not interact negatively with any existing conditions or medications.

Enhancing Livestock Health

In the realm of livestock management, herbal remedies offer a sustainable and natural alternative to conventional medications, reducing the reliance on antibiotics and promoting the overall well-being of the animals. Key applications include:

- Dietary Supplements: Herbs such as garlic and oregano are added to livestock feed as natural antimicrobials and immune boosters.

- Parasite Control: Plants like wormwood and pumpkin seeds are used as natural anthelmintics to control internal parasites.

- Stress Reduction: Adaptogenic herbs, such as ashwagandha, can help manage stress in livestock, particularly during transportation or environmental changes.

Preparation and Use of Herbal Remedies

The preparation of herbal remedies for animals follows principles similar to those for humans but with special consideration for the animal's taste, digestive system, and metabolism. Common preparations include:

- Herbal Teas and Infusions: Easily prepared and administered, herbal teas can be used for a variety of conditions. For example, peppermint tea can aid in digestion, while calendula tea can be used for skin irritations.

- Tinctures and Extracts: Alcohol-based tinctures are generally avoided in animal care. Instead, glycerin-based extracts are used, offering a safe and effective way to administer concentrated herbal remedies.

- Topical Applications: Salves, balms, and poultices made from herbs can be applied directly to the skin to treat wounds, bites, and other external conditions.

Safety and Ethics in Herbalism for Animals

Ensuring the safe use of herbal remedies in animals is paramount. This involves:

- Professional Guidance: Always consult with a veterinarian or a qualified veterinary herbalist before introducing any herbal remedy, especially for animals with pre-existing conditions or those on medication.

- Quality Control: Use high-quality, organic herbs to avoid exposing animals to pesticides and other harmful chemicals.

- Ethical Considerations: Respect for animal welfare and the ethical sourcing of herbs are essential. Sustainable and humane practices should be prioritized to protect both animal health and the environment.

Incorporating herbalism into animal care offers a natural and effective way to enhance the health and well-being of pets and livestock. By understanding the principles of veterinary herbal medicine, recognizing the importance of safety and ethics, and learning how to prepare and use herbal remedies, pet owners and farmers can provide their animals with the benefits of plant-based healing. This approach not only supports the physical health of animals but also contributes to a more sustainable and holistic system of animal care.

Veterinary Herbal Medicine: Use of herbs in treating animal health conditions.

Veterinary herbal medicine harnesses the natural healing power of plants to treat and prevent health conditions in animals. This approach, deeply rooted in the tradition of herbalism, offers a complementary or alternative option to conventional veterinary treatments. It emphasizes the use of whole plants and natural extracts to support the health and well-being of pets and livestock, aligning with a holistic view of animal care.

Selection and Use of Herbs in Veterinary Medicine

The selection of herbs for veterinary use is guided by principles similar to those in human herbalism, but with considerations unique to different animal species. Here are some commonly used herbs and their applications:

- Chamomile: Known for its calming effects, chamomile is often used to relieve stress and anxiety in pets. It can also soothe gastrointestinal upset.

- Ginger: This root is beneficial for nausea and digestive issues in animals, just as it is in humans. It's particularly useful for pets during travel.

- Turmeric: With its potent anti-inflammatory properties, turmeric is used to support joint health and reduce inflammation in animals suffering from conditions like arthritis.

- Milk Thistle: This herb is renowned for its liver-supportive properties and is often recommended for animals with liver conditions or those needing detoxification support.

- Echinacea: Used to boost the immune system, Echinacea can help animals fight off infections and recover more quickly from illness.

Dosage and Administration

Determining the correct dosage is crucial for the safety and effectiveness of herbal treatments in animals. Factors such as the animal's weight, age, species, and overall health condition play a significant role in dosage determination. Herbal remedies can be administered in various forms, including:

- Oral Supplements: Capsules, powders, or liquids mixed with food or given directly.

- Topical Applications: Salves, balms, or poultices applied to the skin for wounds, rashes, or inflammation.

- Herbal Teas: Mild infusions used for gentle internal support or for topical applications in baths or washes.

Safety Considerations

While many herbs are safe for animals, it's essential to proceed with caution. Some plants may be toxic to certain species, or specific parts of a plant could be harmful. For example, the essential oil of tea tree can be toxic to cats when used improperly. Always consult with a veterinary herbalist or a veterinarian knowledgeable in herbal medicine before introducing any new herbal treatment to ensure it's safe and appropriate for your pet or livestock animal.

Integrating Herbal Medicine into Veterinary Care

Integrating herbal medicine into veterinary care requires a collaborative approach. Open communication with a veterinarian ensures that herbal treatments complement conventional care, avoiding any potential interactions with medications or other treatments. Many veterinarians are now recognizing the value of this integrative approach and are either incorporating herbal medicine into their practice or working closely with veterinary herbalists.

The Future of Veterinary Herbal Medicine

As interest in natural and holistic care grows among pet owners and livestock managers, veterinary herbal medicine is poised for expansion. Ongoing research into the efficacy and safety of herbal treatments in animals will further integrate herbalism into veterinary practices, offering a broader range of treatment options for animal health conditions.

Veterinary herbal medicine represents a promising and expanding field, providing natural options for enhancing animal health and well-being. By respecting the principles of herbalism and working closely with veterinary professionals, pet owners and farmers can utilize the healing power of plants to support their animals' health in a holistic and informed manner.

Enhancing Livestock Health: Herbal remedies for common livestock ailments.

Livestock health is paramount for farmers and animal caretakers who rely on these animals for their livelihoods and sustenance. Herbal remedies offer a natural, cost-effective way to support livestock health, treat common ailments, and reduce reliance on synthetic medications, which can lead to resistance and residues in animal products. Here, we explore several herbal remedies known for their efficacy in treating common livestock ailments, emphasizing the importance of integrating these practices with conventional veterinary care.

• Garlic (Allium sativum): Garlic is renowned for its broad-spectrum antimicrobial properties, making it effective against respiratory infections and internal parasites. Incorporating crushed garlic into feed can help deter flies and other pests, promoting a healthier environment for livestock.

• Echinacea (Echinacea spp.): This herb boosts the immune system, making it beneficial during recovery from illness or as a preventive measure during seasonal changes when animals are more susceptible to infections. Echinacea can be added to water or feed in powdered form.

• Peppermint (Mentha piperita): Peppermint is not only refreshing but also has antispasmodic properties, making it useful for digestive issues such as bloating and gas in livestock. A peppermint tea can be prepared and added to drinking water to ease digestive discomfort.

• Chamomile (Matricaria chamomilla): Known for its calming effects, chamomile can be used to reduce stress in animals, especially during transportation or when introducing new animals into a herd. It can also treat minor skin irritations when applied topically as a wash.

• Thyme (Thymus vulgaris): Thyme has strong antiseptic properties, making it useful for respiratory conditions. It can be administered as a tea in drinking water to help alleviate coughs and infections.

• Yarrow (Achillea millefolium): Yarrow is known for its ability to stop bleeding and is useful in treating external wounds. A poultice made from yarrow leaves can be applied directly to cuts and abrasions to promote healing.

• Fennel (Foeniculum vulgare): Fennel is beneficial for its anti-inflammatory and antispasmodic properties, particularly in cases of bloating and gas. Fennel seeds can be mixed into feed to aid digestion and promote overall gut health.

Integrating Herbal Remedies into Livestock Care

When integrating herbal remedies into livestock care, it's crucial to consider the specific needs and conditions of the animals. Start with small doses to ensure there are no adverse reactions and consult with a veterinary herbalist or a veterinarian who is knowledgeable about herbal medicine. Keep detailed records of treatments and outcomes to monitor effectiveness and adjust dosages as needed.

Safety and Quality Control

Ensure the herbs used are of high quality, free from pesticides and contaminants, and correctly identified. Misidentification and contamination can lead to ineffective or harmful treatments. Always source herbs from reputable suppliers and, when possible, grow your own to ensure purity and potency.

Conclusion

Herbal remedies can play a significant role in enhancing livestock health, offering natural solutions for common ailments. By incorporating these practices thoughtfully and safely, farmers and animal caretakers can support the well-being of their livestock, reduce reliance on synthetic medications, and promote a more sustainable approach to animal health care.

CHAPTER 11: HERBALISM AND ENVIRONMENTAL HEALTH

Herbalism extends beyond the personal health benefits it offers, playing a crucial role in promoting environmental health. The interconnectedness of herbal practices and the environment underscores the importance of sustainable approaches to herbalism. This chapter delves into the significance of plants as bioindicators and the pivotal role of biodiversity in effective herbalism, highlighting how these elements contribute to a healthier planet.

Plants as Bioindicators

Plants are nature's sentinels, offering clear signals about the health of our environment. Their sensitivity to changes in soil, air, and water quality makes them excellent bioindicators, helping us detect environmental stresses early. For instance, the presence of certain mosses and lichens can indicate air purity, while the health of aquatic plants reflects water quality. Herbalists and environmentalists alike can use these indicators to monitor and advocate for cleaner, healthier ecosystems.

• Mosses: Known for their sensitivity to air pollutants, mosses can reveal the levels of heavy metals and other toxins in the environment.

• Lichens: These symbiotic organisms are highly sensitive to sulfur dioxide and other air pollutants, making them reliable indicators of air quality.

• Aquatic Plants: The condition of plants in rivers, lakes, and wetlands can indicate water pollution levels, including nutrient overload and toxic substances.

Understanding and observing these natural indicators allow herbalists to choose healthier, less contaminated areas for wildcrafting herbs, ensuring both the potency of remedies and the preservation of the environment.

Herbal Remedies and Biodiversity

Biodiversity is the foundation upon which herbalism stands. The variety of plant species available not only enriches the pharmacopeia of herbal medicine but also supports the resilience of ecosystems. Each plant plays a role in its habitat, contributing to soil health, water regulation, and the balance of oxygen and carbon dioxide in the atmosphere. By valuing and protecting biodiversity, herbalists contribute to the overall health of the planet.

• Soil Health: Diverse plant life contributes to the structure and nutrient content of soil, making it fertile and robust against erosion.

• Water Regulation: Plants play a crucial role in the water cycle, with forests acting as massive sponges that absorb and release water gradually, reducing the risk of floods and droughts.

• Climate Regulation: Through photosynthesis, plants absorb carbon dioxide—a greenhouse gas—thereby mitigating climate change.

Promoting and practicing biodiversity in herbalism involves using a wide range of plant species, supporting local and indigenous plant varieties, and advocating for the conservation of natural habitats. Herbalists can take an active role in biodiversity conservation by:

- Participating in seed exchange programs to preserve plant genetic diversity.

- Supporting conservation efforts and protected areas that safeguard plant species.

- Educating others about the importance of biodiversity for environmental health and herbal medicine.

Sustainable Herbalism Practices

Sustainable harvesting and cultivation practices are essential for maintaining the health of the environment and ensuring the longevity of herbal medicine traditions. Ethical harvesting respects the growth cycles of plants, ensuring that they can regenerate and continue to thrive. Cultivating medicinal herbs, especially those that are endangered or overharvested in the wild, reduces pressure on natural populations and contributes to biodiversity.

- Ethical Wildcrafting: Follow guidelines for sustainable harvesting, such as taking only what you need, leaving plenty of plants behind for regeneration, and harvesting in a way that does not damage the plant or its habitat.

- Organic Cultivation: Grow medicinal herbs using organic methods that enhance soil health and avoid the use of synthetic pesticides and fertilizers, which can harm wildlife and pollute waterways.

- Habitat Restoration: Participate in or support projects that restore habitats, especially those that are crucial for the growth of medicinal plants, enhancing ecosystem health and resilience.

Conclusion

The practice of herbalism is deeply intertwined with environmental health. By understanding and utilizing plants as bioindicators, advocating for biodiversity, and adhering to sustainable practices, herbalists play a vital role in promoting the health of our planet. These efforts not only ensure the efficacy and safety of herbal remedies but also contribute to a legacy of environmental stewardship that will benefit future generations.

Plants as Bioindicators

Plants, including a wide array of herbs, serve as vital bioindicators, offering insightful glimpses into the health of our environment. Their unique ability to respond to changes in their surroundings makes them excellent monitors for assessing the quality of air, water, and soil. By observing these natural indicators, herbalists, gardeners, and environmentalists can gain valuable information about the presence of pollutants and the overall ecological balance of a particular area.

Mosses and lichens, for example, are particularly sensitive to air quality. Their presence or absence in an area can reveal much about the level of air pollution. Mosses tend to accumulate heavy metals, making them reliable indicators of industrial pollution. Lichens, on the other hand, are sensitive to sulfur dioxide and nitrogen oxides, common byproducts of fossil fuel combustion. A decline in lichen diversity or abundance often signals increased air pollution.

Aquatic plants also play a crucial role as bioindicators. The health and variety of plant life in rivers, lakes, and wetlands can provide insights into water quality. Excessive growth of certain algae, for instance, may indicate nutrient pollution from agricultural runoff or sewage discharge. Conversely, the presence of diverse and thriving aquatic plant communities often signifies clean and healthy water bodies.

Herbalists can utilize this knowledge in several ways:

- Site Selection for Wildcrafting: Choosing areas with a rich diversity of mosses, lichens, and healthy aquatic plants can lead to the collection of herbs from less polluted, more vibrant environments.

- Monitoring Environmental Health: Regular observation of local plant life can help track changes in environmental quality over time. This can be especially useful for those who cultivate herbs, as it provides insights into the health of the ecosystem supporting their plants.

- Advocacy and Education: Understanding the role of plants as bioindicators empowers herbalists and environmental enthusiasts to advocate for cleaner, healthier ecosystems. Sharing knowledge about the link between plant health and environmental quality can raise awareness and inspire community action towards sustainability.

To effectively use herbs as bioindicators, consider the following steps:

1. Learn to Identify Local Plants: Familiarize yourself with the mosses, lichens, and aquatic plants in your area. Identification guides and local botanical societies can be valuable resources.

2. Observe and Record: Keep a journal of your observations, noting the types of plants you find and their condition. Over time, this record can reveal trends in environmental health.

3. Engage with Community Science Projects: Participate in or initiate projects that monitor environmental health through plant observations. This can amplify the impact of your efforts and contribute valuable data to larger environmental health studies.

By paying close attention to the plants around us and understanding their role as bioindicators, we can gain insights into the health of our environment and take steps to protect and improve it. This approach not only enriches our practice of herbalism but also contributes to the broader goal of environmental stewardship and sustainability.

Herbal Remedies and Biodiversity

The vitality of plant diversity cannot be overstated in the realm of herbalism. Biodiversity, the variety of life in the world or in a particular habitat or ecosystem, is a cornerstone for the efficacy and sustainability of herbal remedies. The rich tapestry of plant species offers a broad pharmacopeia from which herbalists can draw to treat a wide range of health conditions. This diversity is not just a boon for the herbalist's toolkit; it is essential for the resilience of ecosystems and the plants themselves, offering a buffer against pests, diseases, and changing climate conditions.

• Genetic Diversity Ensures Resilience: Just as a diverse investment portfolio spreads risk, ecological diversity spreads and minimizes environmental threats to plants. This diversity ensures that some species will naturally possess traits allowing them to withstand specific challenges, ensuring the survival of the ecosystem as a whole. For herbalism, this means a more reliable supply of medicinal plants, even as conditions change.

• Wide Range of Medicinal Properties: Different plants have evolved unique chemical compounds as defenses against predators, infections, and diseases. These compounds, in turn, offer a wide range of medicinal properties for human use. The greater the biodiversity, the broader the spectrum of available medicinal compounds, allowing herbalists to tailor treatments more specifically to individual needs.

• Ecosystem Services Support Herbalism: Biodiverse ecosystems provide invaluable services that support the growth and potency of medicinal plants. These include pollination by insects, birds, and bats; soil formation and fertility; nutrient cycling; and water filtration. The loss of biodiversity can disrupt these services, diminishing the quality and availability of medicinal herbs.

To support biodiversity in herbalism, consider the following practices:

- Ethical Wildcrafting: Practice sustainable harvesting techniques that allow plant populations to regenerate. Harvest only what you need and do so in a way that does not harm the plant's long-term survival. This includes being mindful of not overharvesting and avoiding rare or endangered species altogether.

- Cultivate Medicinal Plants: Growing your own herbs not only ensures a sustainable supply but can also contribute to biodiversity, especially if you include a variety of species and heirloom varieties in your garden. This practice supports local wildlife and insect populations, including pollinators crucial for many food crops.

- Support Conservation Efforts: Engage with and support organizations and initiatives aimed at preserving natural habitats and endangered plant species. This can include participating in seed saving and exchange programs, contributing to local and global conservation funds, and advocating for policies that protect natural ecosystems.

- Educate and Spread Awareness: Share knowledge about the importance of biodiversity in herbalism with your community. Education can inspire others to adopt practices that support ecological health, creating a larger impact on conservation efforts.

In essence, the relationship between herbalism and biodiversity is symbiotic. By fostering and maintaining the diversity of plant life, herbalists ensure not only the efficacy and sustainability of their practices but also contribute to the health of the planet. This mutual support system underscores the importance of conservation efforts and sustainable practices within the herbalism community, ensuring that the ancient art of herbal healing can continue to flourish for generations to come.

CHAPTER 12: ADVANCED HERBAL PREPARATION TECHNIQUES

Fermentation and Herbal Brews

Fermentation is a transformative process that not only preserves herbs but also enhances their medicinal properties. This ancient technique involves the breakdown of a substance by bacteria, yeasts, or other microorganisms, resulting in a product that is rich in probiotics, enzymes, and vitamins. Here's how to create probiotic-rich herbal beverages:

1. Select Your Herbs: Choose herbs known for their digestive benefits, such as peppermint, ginger, or chamomile.

2. Prepare a Sweet Tea: Brew a strong herbal tea as the base for your fermentation. Sweeten with honey or sugar, which will serve as food for the fermenting bacteria.

3. Cool and Combine: Once the tea has cooled to room temperature, transfer it to a fermentation vessel. Add a starter culture, such as a SCOBY (Symbiotic Culture Of Bacteria and Yeast) for kombucha or whey for herbal kefir.

4. Ferment: Cover the vessel with a breathable cloth to prevent contaminants while allowing air to circulate. Store in a warm, dark place for a period ranging from a few days to several weeks, depending on the desired strength of fermentation.

5. Bottle and Refrigerate: Once fermentation is complete, bottle your brew, leaving some space at the top for gases. Store in the refrigerator to slow further fermentation.

★☆☆☆☆ Difficulty: Easy to moderate, depending on your familiarity with fermentation.

Advanced Extraction Methods

Maximizing the potency of herbal extracts often involves techniques that go beyond simple infusion or decoction. Here are methods to extract the most medicinal compounds from your herbs:

1. Percolation: This method is akin to making coffee, where water or alcohol drips through a column of finely ground herbs, extracting their medicinal properties more efficiently than simple steeping.

   - Grind your herbs to a fine consistency.

   - Moisten the herbs with a portion of your solvent (water or alcohol) to create a "magma."

   - Pack the magma into a percolation cone (a glass or stainless steel column).

   - Slowly pour your solvent over the packed herbs, collecting the extract from the bottom of the cone.

2. Soxhlet Extraction: This technique requires specialized equipment but is highly effective in extracting soluble compounds using a continuous cycle of solvent evaporation and condensation.

   - Place your herbs in the extraction chamber of the Soxhlet apparatus.

   - Fill the round-bottom flask with your solvent and heat it to boil.

   - The solvent vapors will ascend, condense, and then percolate through the herbs, extracting their compounds before being recycled back into the flask.

3. Supercritical Fluid Extraction (SFE): This advanced method uses supercritical CO_2 as the solvent. It's highly efficient and yields pure extracts without solvent residues, but it requires specialized equipment.

   - The CO_2 is pressurized and heated until it reaches a supercritical state, where it has properties of both a gas and a liquid.

   - This supercritical CO_2 is then passed through the herbs, dissolving the desired compounds.

   - After extraction, the CO_2 is depressurized, returning it to a gas and leaving behind the pure extract.

$$$$$ Cost Estimate: High, due to the need for specialized equipment, especially for Soxhlet and SFE methods.

√ Safety Tips:

- Always follow safety guidelines when handling solvents, especially flammable ones like alcohol.

- Ensure proper ventilation when using heat and solvents.

- Wear protective gear, including gloves and goggles, when handling concentrated extracts.

By incorporating these advanced herbal preparation techniques into your practice, you can enhance the efficacy and shelf-life of your herbal remedies. Whether you're fermenting herbal brews to create probiotic-rich drinks or using sophisticated extraction methods to concentrate the medicinal properties of plants, these techniques represent the cutting edge of herbalism, offering potent ways to harness the healing power of nature.

Fermentation and Herbal Brews: Creating probiotic-rich herbal beverages.

Fermentation is a revered process in the realm of herbalism, transforming simple herbal teas into probiotic-rich beverages that offer a myriad of health benefits. This method not only preserves the herbs but also amplifies their medicinal qualities, making it a valuable technique for anyone interested in natural health remedies. Here's how to embark on the journey of creating your own fermented herbal brews.

1. Select Your Herbs: Begin by choosing herbs that are beneficial for digestion and overall health. Peppermint, ginger, and chamomile are excellent choices due to their soothing properties. Each herb brings its unique benefits to the brew, enhancing the flavor and health properties of the final product.

2. Prepare a Sweet Tea: Brew a strong herbal tea using your selected herbs. This will serve as the base for your fermentation. To feed the fermenting bacteria, sweeten the tea with natural sweeteners like honey or sugar. Ensure the tea is well-dissolved and mixed.

3. Cool and Combine: Allow the sweetened herbal tea to cool to room temperature. This is crucial to avoid killing the starter culture with excessive heat. Once cooled, transfer the tea into a clean fermentation vessel. Add your starter culture to the vessel; this could be a SCOBY (for kombucha) or whey (for kefir), depending on the type of fermented drink you're aiming to create.

4. Ferment: Cover the vessel with a breathable cloth to keep out unwanted particles while allowing air to circulate, which is essential for fermentation. Place the vessel in a warm, dark place—a cupboard or pantry works well. The fermentation process can take anywhere from a few days to several weeks, depending on the temperature and the strength you desire.

5. Bottle and Refrigerate: After fermentation has reached its desired level, it's time to bottle your brew. Use clean bottles and leave some space at the top to accommodate any gases that may form. Seal the bottles and store them in the refrigerator to halt the fermentation process. This will preserve the flavor and probiotic content of your herbal brew.

★☆☆☆☆ Difficulty: This process is relatively easy, even for beginners in fermentation. The key is patience and attention to the cleanliness of your tools and workspace.

Creating fermented herbal brews is not only a way to enjoy the health benefits of herbs but also a delightful exploration into the ancient art of fermentation. Each batch is unique, and with practice, you can tailor the flavors and medicinal properties to suit your preferences and health needs. Enjoy the process and the delicious, healthful drinks you create, knowing you're partaking in a timeless tradition of herbal healing.

Advanced Extraction Methods: Techniques for maximizing the potency of herbal extracts.

To maximize the potency of herbal extracts, advanced extraction methods can be employed to isolate and concentrate the active compounds found in medicinal plants. These techniques, while more complex, offer a higher yield and purity of the desired constituents, making the extracts more effective for therapeutic use. Here are some of the advanced methods used in herbal extraction:

1. Ultrasonic Extraction: This method uses ultrasonic waves to create small vibrations within the plant material. These vibrations break down the cell walls, allowing the active compounds to be released into the solvent more efficiently.

- Fill an ultrasonic extractor with your solvent and add the plant material.

- Set the timer and temperature according to the herb and compound you wish to extract.

- Once the extraction is complete, filter the mixture to separate the liquid extract from the plant material.

2. Microwave-Assisted Extraction: Microwave energy is used to heat the solvent and plant material mixture, speeding up the extraction process and improving the extraction yield.

- Combine the plant material and solvent in a microwave-safe container.

- Microwave at a specified power and time, taking care not to overheat and degrade the active compounds.

- Cool the mixture before filtering to obtain the extract.

3. Enzyme-Assisted Extraction: This method involves using enzymes to break down the cell walls of the plant material, making it easier for the solvent to extract the active compounds.

- Select enzymes that target the specific cell wall components of your plant material.

- Mix the plant material with the enzymes and a suitable solvent, and incubate at the recommended temperature.

- After incubation, filter the mixture to collect the extract.

4. Supercritical CO2 Extraction: This technique uses supercritical carbon dioxide as the solvent. At supercritical conditions, CO2 has both gas and liquid properties, allowing it to penetrate plant material and dissolve compounds more effectively.

- Place the plant material in the extraction chamber of a supercritical CO2 extractor.

- Bring the CO2 to a supercritical state by adjusting the temperature and pressure settings.

- After extraction, depressurize the system to separate the extract from the CO2.

5. Counter-Current Extraction: This continuous method involves passing the solvent through a series of vessels containing the plant material in the opposite direction. It's particularly effective for extracting compounds from large quantities of plant material.

- Arrange the extraction vessels in a series, with each vessel connected to the next.

- Add the plant material to each vessel and start the flow of solvent from the last vessel to the first.

- Collect the extract from the first vessel, which will contain the highest concentration of the desired compounds.

√ Safety Tips:

- Always wear protective equipment, including gloves and goggles, when handling solvents and plant materials.

- Ensure adequate ventilation in the extraction area to avoid inhalation of harmful vapors.

- Be familiar with the operating procedures and safety features of the extraction equipment.

$$$$$ Cost Estimate: The cost of these advanced extraction methods can vary widely, with supercritical CO2 extraction and microwave-assisted extraction being among the more expensive options due to the specialized equipment required. However, the investment can be justified by the higher quality and potency of the extracts produced.

By employing these advanced extraction techniques, herbalists and manufacturers can produce highly potent herbal extracts. These concentrated forms of the plant's active compounds offer enhanced therapeutic benefits, making them valuable for a wide range of health applications.

CHAPTER 13: THE PSYCHOLOGICAL EFFECTS OF HERBALISM

The psychological effects of herbalism extend far beyond the physical benefits of the herbs themselves, influencing mental health, emotional well-being, and overall life satisfaction. Engaging with herbalism can have profound impacts on one's psychological state, offering a sense of connection, empowerment, and tranquility that is often overlooked in conventional medicine.

The Placebo Effect and Herbalism

The placebo effect plays a significant role in the psychological impact of herbal treatments. This phenomenon occurs when a person experiences a real alteration in their condition after receiving a treatment that has no therapeutic effect on the targeted ailment. In herbalism, the belief in the healing power of plants can enhance the efficacy of treatments through the placebo effect, demonstrating the intricate connection between mind and body.

• Expectation and Healing: The anticipation of positive outcomes can trigger physiological responses that contribute to healing. Engaging with herbal remedies often comes with the expectation of relief, which can initiate a healing process in the body.

• Ritual and Routine: The process of preparing and using herbal remedies creates a ritualistic practice that can offer psychological comfort and stability, further enhancing the placebo effect.

Emotional Well-being and Plant Interaction

Interacting with plants, whether through gardening, wildcrafting, or simply being in nature, has been shown to improve mood, reduce stress, and enhance overall emotional well-being. The act of caring for plants and engaging with the natural world can ground individuals, offering a sense of peace and fulfillment.

• Stress Reduction: Activities like gardening or preparing herbal remedies can act as a form of mindfulness practice, focusing the mind on the present moment and alleviating stress.

• Connection to Nature: Herbalism fosters a deep connection with the natural world, promoting a sense of belonging and an appreciation for the cycle of life. This connection can combat feelings of isolation and promote a sense of community and interdependence.

Psychological Empowerment through Herbalism

Learning about and practicing herbalism can lead to psychological empowerment. Gaining knowledge and skills in identifying, harvesting, and preparing herbal remedies provides individuals with a sense of autonomy over their health and well-being.

• Self-Efficacy: The ability to care for oneself and loved ones with natural remedies boosts confidence and self-reliance, contributing to a stronger sense of self-efficacy.

• Knowledge Sharing: Sharing herbal knowledge and practices with others can enhance social bonds and provide a sense of purpose and contribution to the community.

Mindfulness and Herbal Practices

The preparation and use of herbal remedies require attention to detail, patience, and mindfulness. These practices can help individuals develop a more mindful approach to life, appreciating the small details and finding joy in the process.

• Presence in the Moment: The tactile experience of handling herbs, the aromas, and the process of creating remedies can help anchor individuals in the present moment, reducing anxiety and promoting mental clarity.

• Meditative Practices: Many find the process of preparing herbal remedies to be meditative, offering a peaceful retreat from the hustle and bustle of daily life.

Conclusion

The psychological effects of herbalism are multifaceted, offering benefits that extend well beyond the physical healing properties of plants. Through the placebo effect, emotional well-being, psychological empowerment, and mindfulness, engaging with herbalism can provide a holistic approach to health that nurtures the mind, body, and spirit. As individuals explore the ancient art of herbal healing, they may discover not only a deeper connection to the natural world but also an enhanced sense of peace, purpose, and joy in their lives.

The Placebo Effect and Herbalism

The placebo effect, a fascinating and often misunderstood phenomenon, plays a crucial role in the realm of herbalism, shedding light on the profound psychological impact of herbal treatments. At its core, the placebo effect occurs when individuals experience a tangible improvement in their health or symptoms after receiving a treatment that has no active therapeutic effect on the condition being treated. This effect underscores the powerful interplay between the mind and body, revealing that the belief in the efficacy of a treatment can significantly influence one's physical health.

Herbal treatments, with their rich history and cultural significance, are particularly conducive to eliciting a strong placebo response. The act of taking an herbal remedy, often steeped in traditional practices and rituals, can enhance an individual's expectation of healing, thereby activating the placebo effect. This expectation triggers a series of biochemical processes in the brain that can lead to real physiological changes, such as the release of endorphins and other natural painkillers, which can alleviate symptoms and promote well-being.

Moreover, the sensory experiences associated with herbal remedies—such as their taste, smell, and the tactile act of preparing them—can further reinforce the expectation of benefit, making the placebo effect more pronounced. For instance, the calming aroma of lavender or the soothing taste of chamomile tea can enhance an individual's psychological and physiological response to the treatment, beyond the herbs' intrinsic properties.

The ritualistic aspect of herbalism also contributes significantly to the placebo effect. The deliberate and mindful preparation of herbal remedies, from selecting and measuring herbs to brewing teas or compounding salves, can create a therapeutic ritual that promotes a sense of control over one's health and well-being. This ritualistic engagement not only fosters a deeper connection to the healing process but also amplifies the placebo effect by instilling confidence and optimism in the efficacy of the treatment.

Furthermore, the social and cultural context in which herbal remedies are used can influence the strength of the placebo effect. In communities where herbalism is a respected and integral part of health care, the collective belief in the power of herbs can enhance the individual's expectation of healing, thereby magnifying the placebo response. This collective belief system, passed down through generations, adds a layer of psychological support that bolsters the individual's confidence in the treatment and its potential benefits.

In understanding the placebo effect within herbalism, it becomes clear that the psychological impact of herbal treatments is a critical component of their efficacy. This effect highlights the importance of considering the holistic experience of herbal therapy, including the psychological, cultural, and sensory factors that contribute to healing. By acknowledging and embracing the placebo effect, herbalists and practitioners can enhance the therapeutic potential of herbal remedies, offering a more comprehensive and effective approach to health and wellness that bridges the gap between mind and body.

Emotional Well-being and Plant Interaction

Engaging with plants and immersing oneself in the natural world has profound effects on emotional well-being and mental health. This connection, deeply rooted in our evolutionary past, offers a respite from the fast-paced digital world, grounding us in the present moment and providing a sense of peace and tranquility.

The act of caring for plants, whether indoors or in a garden, can be a meditative and therapeutic practice. It encourages mindfulness, a state of active, open attention to the present. This mindfulness can reduce stress, anxiety, and symptoms of depression. The simple routine of watering, pruning, and tending to plants can establish a daily ritual of care that fosters a sense of responsibility, achievement, and satisfaction.

Moreover, the presence of plants in one's living or working environment can improve air quality and increase feelings of vitality and energy. Studies have shown that indoor plants can reduce fatigue, coughs, sore throats, and other cold-related illnesses by more than

30%, primarily due to their effects on indoor humidity levels and air purification.

Gardening, as a form of physical exercise, can also contribute to improved mental health. It offers exposure to vitamin D, increases levels of physical activity, and can lead to improved sleep patterns and better overall health. The act of growing one's food can also contribute to a sense of accomplishment and can improve one's diet, further enhancing mental health.

The psychological benefits of plant interaction are not limited to individual experiences. Community gardens and green spaces foster social interaction, create a sense of community, and can reduce loneliness among diverse groups of people, including the elderly, immigrants, and those with mental health conditions.

Incorporating plant care into daily life doesn't require a large garden or extensive knowledge of horticulture. Starting small with a few indoor plants or herbs can be just as beneficial. Here are some simple steps to begin integrating plants into your life for improved mental health:

1. Choose low-maintenance plants: Start with plants that are easy to care for and resilient, such as succulents, snake plants, or spider plants.

2. Create a routine: Incorporate plant care into your daily or weekly routine. This could be a set time for watering, pruning, or simply checking on your plants.

3. Connect with community: Join a local gardening club or community garden. This can provide valuable knowledge and a sense of belonging.

4. Mindfulness practice: Use time with your plants to practice mindfulness. Observe the colors, textures, and growth of your plants without judgment.

5. Educate yourself: Learn about the plants you are caring for. Understanding their needs and growth patterns can make the experience more rewarding.

By fostering a connection with plants, individuals can tap into the calming and restorative powers of nature, enhancing their emotional well-being and mental health. This interaction is a testament to the timeless wisdom of herbalism and its potential to transform modern health and wellness, offering a natural and accessible tool for improving quality of life.

HERBAL REMEDIES

Gut-Healing Broth

Ingredients:

- 4 quarts filtered water
- 2 pounds of mixed organic, grass-fed beef bones (knuckles and marrow bones)
- 2 carrots, chopped
- 2 celery stalks, chopped
- 1 onion, chopped
- 2 cloves of garlic, smashed
- 1 teaspoon of Himalayan pink salt
- 1 teaspoon of apple cider vinegar
- A handful of fresh parsley
- 2 bay leaves
- ½ teaspoon of whole peppercorns

Instructions:

1. Place all ingredients except for parsley in a large stockpot or slow cooker.

2. Bring to a boil, then reduce heat to simmer. For a stockpot, simmer for 24-48 hours; for a slow cooker, set to low for the same duration.

3. During the last 30 minutes of cooking, add the fresh parsley.

4. Strain the broth through a fine mesh sieve, discarding the solids.

5. Allow the broth to cool, and then store in glass containers in the refrigerator for up to 5 days or freeze for up to 3 months.

Portions: Makes approximately 4 servings.

Beneficial Effects: This broth is designed to soothe the digestive tract, reduce inflammation, and rebuild the gut lining. It provides essential nutrients for gut repair, including collagen, amino acids, minerals, and vitamins.

Root Cause of Illness: Compromised gut health due to poor diet, stress, and antibiotics leading to issues such as leaky gut syndrome, inflammation, and digestive discomfort.

Tips for Allergens: Ensure all ingredients are organic to minimize exposure to pesticides and herbicides. For individuals sensitive to histamines, reduce cooking time to 6-8 hours, and consume fresh or freeze immediately to prevent histamine build-up.

This recipe, rooted in Barbara O'Neill's theory, emphasizes the importance of natural, whole-food ingredients for addressing and preventing digestive health issues. The inclusion of apple cider vinegar aids in the extraction of minerals from the bones, enhancing the broth's nutritional profile.

Gentle Digestive Biscuits

Ingredients:

- 1 cup whole wheat flour (for fiber content)
- 1/2 cup rolled oats (rich in beta-glucan, a soluble fiber)
- 1/4 cup ground flaxseed (for Omega-3 fatty acids and fiber)
- 1/4 cup almond milk (or any plant-based milk)
- 1/4 cup coconut oil (for healthy fats)
- 2 tablespoons honey (natural sweetener)
- 1 teaspoon ground ginger (for soothing the stomach)
- 1/2 teaspoon baking powder (aluminum-free)
- A pinch of salt (preferably Himalayan pink salt)

Instructions:

6. Preheat your oven to 350°F (177°C).

7. In a large mixing bowl, combine the whole wheat flour, rolled oats, ground flaxseed, ginger, baking powder, and salt.

8. Melt the coconut oil and mix it with almond milk and honey in a separate bowl.

9. Combine the wet and dry ingredients until a cohesive dough forms.

10. Roll the dough into small balls and flatten them slightly to form biscuits. Place them on a baking sheet lined with parchment paper.

11. Bake for 12-15 minutes or until the edges are golden brown.

12. Allow the biscuits to cool on a wire rack before serving.

Portions: Makes approximately 20 biscuits.

Beneficial Effects: These biscuits are designed to promote digestive wellness through the gentle stimulation of digestive processes, aiding in the relief of constipation and the promotion of regular bowel movements. The inclusion of dietary fiber supports a healthy gut microbiome, while the calming properties of ingredients like ginger and peppermint can soothe stomach discomfort.

Root Cause of Illness: Digestive discomfort and irregularities often stem from insufficient fiber intake, overconsumption of processed foods, and a lack of essential nutrients that support gut health.

Tips for Allergens:

Ensure all ingredients are certified gluten-free if necessary.

For a nut-free version, substitute almond milk with oat milk or any other preferred plant-based milk that does not contain nuts.

Always check labels for potential cross-contamination if you have severe allergies.

Portion Control: One to two biscuits per serving are recommended. Overconsumption may lead to excessive fiber intake, which can cause digestive discomfort for some individuals.

Storage: Store in an airtight container at room temperature for up to 5 days, or refrigerate for extended freshness.

Probiotic Yogurt Delight

Ingredients:

• 2 cups of organic, full-fat plain yogurt (ensure it contains live cultures)
• 1 tablespoon of raw honey (optional, for sweetness)
• ½ cup of fresh berries (blueberries, strawberries, or raspberries for antioxidants)
• 1 tablespoon of ground flaxseeds (for omega-3 fatty acids and fiber)
• 1 teaspoon of vanilla extract (for flavor)

Instructions:

13. In a medium-sized bowl, combine the plain yogurt with the raw honey (if using) and vanilla extract. Stir until well mixed.

14. Gently fold in the fresh berries, ensuring they are evenly distributed throughout the yogurt.

15. Sprinkle the ground flaxseeds over the top of the yogurt mixture.

16. Divide the mixture into two serving bowls or glasses.

17. Serve immediately or refrigerate for 30 minutes before serving if a cooler dessert is preferred.

Portions: Serves 2

Beneficial Effects: Enhances gut health by introducing beneficial probiotics, aids in digestion, and supports a healthy immune system.

Root Cause of Illness: Imbalances in the gut microbiome can lead to various digestive issues, including bloating, indigestion, and irregular bowel movements.

Tips for Allergens: For those with dairy sensitivities, substitute the dairy yogurt with a high-quality, probiotic-rich coconut yogurt or another plant-based yogurt alternative. Always ensure that the substitute contains live cultures for the full probiotic benefit. If opting for honey, ensure it is raw and organic to avoid potential allergens and additives found in processed honey.

Herbal Digestive Tonic

Ingredients:

- 1 tablespoon dried chamomile flowers
- 1 tablespoon dried peppermint leaves
- 1 teaspoon fennel seeds
- 1 teaspoon ginger root, freshly grated
- 2 cups boiling water
- Honey (optional, to taste)

Instructions:

18. In a teapot or heat-resistant glass container, combine the chamomile flowers, peppermint leaves, fennel seeds, and freshly grated ginger root.

19. Pour 2 cups of boiling water over the herbal mixture. Cover and steep for 10-15 minutes to allow the herbs to infuse their properties into the water.

20. Strain the tonic to remove the solid ingredients. Add honey to taste, if desired, for sweetness.

21. Consume the tonic warm. For digestive support, drink 1 cup 20-30 minutes before meals.

Portions: Makes 2 servings.

Beneficial Effects:

Chamomile is known for its calming effects on the digestive system, helping to ease indigestion and soothe stomach aches.

Peppermint aids in relaxing the digestive tract muscles, which can alleviate symptoms of irritable bowel syndrome (IBS) and reduce bloating.

Fennel seeds are effective in combating gas and cramping, promoting overall digestive comfort.

Ginger stimulates digestion, enhances nutrient absorption, and can help to reduce nausea.

Root Cause of Illness: This tonic is designed to address various digestive issues such as indigestion, bloating, gas, and discomfort by harnessing the natural soothing and stimulative properties of the included herbs.

Tips for Allergens:

Individuals with allergies to plants in the Asteraceae family should exercise caution with chamomile due to potential allergic reactions.

Those with a history of gallstones should consult a healthcare provider before consuming ginger.

Peppermint may aggravate symptoms in people with GERD (gastroesophageal reflux disease) or hiatal hernia.

Soothing Aloe Vera Gel

Ingredients:

• 1 large Aloe Vera leaf (to extract 1 cup of pure Aloe Vera gel)
• 1 tablespoon Vitamin E oil (to preserve the gel and add extra nourishing properties)
• Optional: 5 drops of lavender essential oil (for added antimicrobial and soothing effects)

Instructions:

22. Carefully slice the Aloe Vera leaf lengthwise to open it.

23. Use a spoon to scoop out the clear gel inside.

24. Place the gel in a blender, adding the Vitamin E oil and optional lavender essential oil.

25. Blend on high for 30 seconds until the mixture is smooth.

26. Pour the gel into a clean, airtight container.

27. Store in the refrigerator for up to one week.

Portions: Yields approximately 1 cup.

Beneficial Effects: Aloe Vera Gel is renowned for its soothing, moisturizing, and healing properties. It provides a protective barrier that helps keep moisture locked in, soothes irritated skin, reduces inflammation, and promotes faster healing of minor cuts and burns. Its anti-inflammatory and antimicrobial properties also make it beneficial for acne-prone skin.

Root Cause of Illness: Skin irritation and inflammation often stem from environmental factors such as pollution, UV exposure, and harsh chemicals found in many skincare products. These factors can compromise the skin's natural barrier, leading to dryness, redness, and sensitivity.

Tips for Allergens: Ensure the Aloe Vera plant and any added oils are pure and free from contaminants. Individuals with sensitivities to essential oils should perform a patch test before applying widely or omit the essential oil from the recipe.

This Soothing Aloe Vera Gel recipe, based on Barbara O'Neill's holistic health principles, utilizes the natural healing properties of Aloe Vera, enhanced with Vitamin E and optional lavender oil, to provide a gentle and effective remedy for various skin concerns.

Hydrating Cucumber Tonic

Ingredients:

- 1 large cucumber, peeled and sliced
- 2 cups of water
- 1 tablespoon of honey (optional, for sweetness)
- Juice of 1 lemon
- A handful of fresh mint leaves

Instructions:

28. In a blender, combine the cucumber slices and water. Blend until smooth.

29. Strain the cucumber mixture through a fine mesh sieve or cheesecloth into a pitcher, discarding the solids.

30. Stir in the lemon juice and honey (if using) until well combined.

31. Add the fresh mint leaves to the pitcher.

32. Chill in the refrigerator for at least 1 hour before serving.

33. Serve over ice for a refreshing and hydrating tonic.

Portions: Serves 4

Beneficial Effects:

Provides hydration and replenishes electrolytes lost through sweat.

Cucumber and lemon offer detoxifying properties and promote skin health.

Mint aids in digestion and adds a refreshing flavor.

Honey, a natural sweetener, contains antioxidants and can soothe sore throats.

Root Cause of Illness: Dehydration and its impact on overall health, including skin dryness, fatigue, and impaired digestion.

Tips for Allergens:

Ensure the honey is pure and free from additives to avoid potential allergens. For a vegan option, substitute honey with maple syrup.

For those with sensitivities, all ingredients can be adjusted or omitted as necessary to accommodate dietary restrictions.

Celery Seed Extract

Ingredients:

- 1 tablespoon celery seeds
- 1 cup boiling water
- Optional: 1 teaspoon honey or lemon juice for flavor

Instructions:

34. Place the celery seeds in a tea infuser or directly into a cup.

35. Pour 1 cup of boiling water over the seeds.

36. Allow the tea to steep for 10-15 minutes.

37. Remove the tea infuser or strain the tea to remove the seeds.

38. Optional: Add honey or lemon juice to taste, if desired.

Portions: Makes 1 serving.

Beneficial Effects:

Celery seed extract acts as a natural diuretic, supporting kidney health and aiding in the elimination of toxins from the body.

Contains antioxidants that help reduce inflammation, particularly beneficial for those suffering from joint pain or gout.

May help lower blood pressure and cholesterol levels, contributing to overall cardiovascular health.

Root Cause of Illness: Targets inflammation and uric acid buildup in the body, which can lead to joint pain and discomfort.

Tips for Allergens:

Celery seeds are generally safe, but individuals with known allergies to celery should avoid this remedy.

For those with a honey allergy or following a vegan diet, the honey can be omitted or substituted with maple syrup.

Licorice Root Digestive Soothe

Ingredients:

- 1 tablespoon dried licorice root
- 1 cup boiling water
- Optional: 1 teaspoon honey for sweetness

Instructions:

39. Place the dried licorice root in a tea infuser or directly into a cup.

40. Pour 1 cup of boiling water over the licorice root.

41. Allow the tea to steep for 10-15 minutes.

42. Remove the tea infuser or strain the tea to remove the licorice root.

43. Optional: Add honey to taste, if desired.

Portions: Makes 1 serving

Beneficial Effects:

Soothes the digestive tract and relieves symptoms of indigestion and heartburn.

Acts as a mild laxative, aiding in constipation relief.

Supports the repair of the stomach lining and reduces inflammation.

Root Cause of Illness: Targets digestive issues caused by inflammation and irritation of the stomach lining, including acid reflux, heartburn, and constipation.

Tips for Allergens:

Ensure the licorice root is pure and free from cross-contaminants if you have specific food allergies.

Individuals with hypertension should use licorice root sparingly, as it can affect blood pressure levels.

Always consult with a healthcare provider before incorporating herbal remedies into your regimen, especially if you are pregnant, nursing, or on medication.

Probiotic Gut-Brain Axis Balance

Ingredients:

- 1 cup plain, unsweetened yogurt (rich in probiotics)
- 1 tablespoon ground flaxseeds (source of prebiotic fiber)
- 1/2 banana (for natural sweetness and prebiotic benefits)
- 1/4 teaspoon ground cinnamon (for flavor and digestive health)
- 1 tablespoon almond butter (healthy fats and additional fiber)
- 1 teaspoon honey (optional, for sweetness)

Instructions:

44. In a blender, combine the yogurt, ground flaxseeds, banana, cinnamon, and almond butter.

45. Blend until the mixture is smooth and creamy.

46. Taste the mixture and add honey if a sweeter flavor is desired. Blend again briefly to incorporate the honey.

47. Serve the mixture in a bowl or glass. For an added probiotic boost, sprinkle with a small amount of additional ground flaxseeds.

Portions: Serves 1

Beneficial Effects:

Supports the gut-brain axis by enhancing gut health with probiotics, which in turn can positively impact mental clarity and mood.

Ground flaxseeds provide prebiotic fiber, promoting the growth of beneficial gut bacteria.

Almond butter and banana add nutritional value and fiber, further supporting digestive health and providing energy.

Root Cause of Illness: Targets imbalances in the gut microbiome, which can affect mental health and cognitive function due to the interconnected nature of the gut-brain axis.

Tips for Allergens:

For those with dairy sensitivities, substitute plain, unsweetened yogurt with a high-quality, probiotic-rich coconut yogurt or another plant-based yogurt alternative. Ensure that the substitute contains live cultures for the full probiotic benefit.

If opting for honey, ensure it is raw and organic to avoid potential allergens and additives found in processed honey.

GABA Calm Capsules

Ingredients:

- 500 mg GABA (Gamma-Aminobutyric Acid) powder
- 100 mg Magnesium glycinate powder
- 50 mg L-Theanine powder
- Capsule shells (vegetarian or gelatin, as preferred)

Instructions:

48. In a clean, dry mixing bowl, combine GABA, magnesium glycinate, and L-Theanine powders. Mix thoroughly to ensure even distribution of all ingredients.

49. Using a capsule machine or a small spoon, carefully fill each capsule shell with the mixture. Follow the capsule machine's instructions for sealing the capsules.

50. Store the filled capsules in a cool, dry place, away from direct sunlight. Airtight containers are recommended to preserve the potency of the capsules.

Portions: This recipe yields approximately 60 capsules, depending on the size of the capsule shells used.

Beneficial Effects:

GABA serves as a neurotransmitter that helps calm the nervous system, reducing feelings of anxiety and stress.

Magnesium glycinate is known for its ability to promote relaxation and improve sleep quality.

L-Theanine, an amino acid found in green tea, enhances the calming effects of GABA and contributes to improved focus and mental clarity.

Root Cause of Illness: Targets stress and anxiety by modulating neurotransmitter activity in the brain, promoting a sense of calm and relaxation.

Tips for Allergens:

Ensure all ingredients are free from contaminants and allergens. Individuals with specific dietary restrictions should select capsule shells that meet their needs (e.g., vegetarian capsules for those avoiding animal products).

Always consult with a healthcare provider before starting any new supplement regimen, especially if you have underlying health conditions or are taking other medications.

Skullcap Serenity Brew

Ingredients:

- 1 tablespoon dried skullcap herb
- 2 cups boiling water
- Optional: honey or lemon to taste

Instructions:

51. Place the dried skullcap herb in a tea infuser or directly into a cup.

52. Pour 2 cups of boiling water over the skullcap.

53. Allow the tea to steep for 10-15 minutes.

54. Remove the tea infuser or strain the tea to remove the loose herbs.

55. Optional: Add honey or lemon to taste, if desired.

Portions: Makes 2 servings

Beneficial Effects:

Promotes relaxation and reduces stress without causing drowsiness.

Supports the nervous system, aiding in the relief of anxiety and nervous tension.

Encourages healthy sleep patterns, making it beneficial for those with insomnia.

Root Cause of Illness: Targets stress and anxiety by calming the mind and body, addressing the root cause of sleep disturbances and nervous tension.

Tips for Allergens:

Skullcap is generally well-tolerated, but individuals with a history of plant allergies should proceed with caution.

For those with allergies to honey or citrus, these ingredients can be omitted without significantly altering the benefits of the tea.

Kava Kava Muscle Relaxant

Ingredients:

- 1 tablespoon kava kava root powder
- 1 cup hot water (not boiling)
- Optional: honey or lemon to taste

Instructions:

56. Place the kava kava root powder in a bowl.

57. Add 1 cup of hot water to the bowl. Ensure the water is hot but not boiling to preserve the active ingredients in the kava kava.

58. Let the mixture steep for 15 minutes.

59. Strain the liquid using a fine mesh strainer or cheesecloth to remove the kava kava root particles.

60. Optional: Add honey or lemon to taste, if desired.

Portions: Makes 1 serving.

Beneficial Effects:

Promotes relaxation and reduces anxiety without impairing cognitive function.

Supports muscle relaxation and can alleviate symptoms of stress-induced muscle tension.

May improve sleep quality by inducing a state of calmness.

Root Cause of Illness: Targets stress and anxiety by modulating the activity of neurotransmitters associated with the stress response, providing a natural way to relax the mind and body.

Tips for Allergens:

Kava kava is generally considered safe for most individuals, but it is important to consult with a healthcare provider before use, especially for those with liver issues or taking medications that affect the liver.

For those with allergies to honey or citrus, these ingredients can be omitted.

Arnica Montana Bruise Balm

Ingredients:

- 1/2 cup arnica montana flowers (dried)
- 1 cup olive oil (as a base for infusion)
- 1/4 cup beeswax (to thicken the salve)
- Optional: 10 drops of lavender essential oil (for additional anti-inflammatory and soothing effects)

Instructions:

61. Combine the dried arnica flowers with olive oil in a double boiler. Gently heat the mixture over low heat for 2-3 hours to allow the arnica to infuse into the oil.

62. Strain the arnica-infused oil through a cheesecloth or fine mesh strainer to remove the flowers. Discard the flowers and return the infused oil to the double boiler.

63. Add the beeswax to the infused oil and heat gently, stirring until the beeswax is completely melted and combined with the oil.

64. If using, add the lavender essential oil to the mixture and stir well.

65. Carefully pour the hot mixture into small tins or glass jars. Allow to cool and solidify at room temperature.

66. Once cooled, seal the containers. Label with the contents and date.

Portions: Makes about 3/4 cup of Arnica Montana Bruise Balm.

Beneficial Effects:

Provides natural pain relief and reduces inflammation due to the salicin content, which the body converts into salicylic acid, similar to aspirin.

Can help alleviate headaches, menstrual cramps, arthritis, and other types of pain.

Root Cause of Illness: Targets pain and inflammation by inhibiting the production of pain-inducing chemicals in the body.

Tips for Allergens:

Ensure all ingredients are pure and free from contaminants. Individuals with sensitivities to beeswax or lavender should omit these ingredients or substitute with suitable alternatives. Always perform a patch test before applying the salve to larger areas of skin, especially for those with sensitive skin or allergies to botanical ingredients.

Willow Bark Headache Cure

Ingredients:

- 2 tablespoons of dried white willow bark
- 4 cups of water
- Optional: Honey or lemon to taste

Instructions:

67. In a medium saucepan, bring the water to a boil.

68. Add the dried white willow bark to the boiling water.

69. Reduce the heat and simmer for 20 minutes.

70. Remove from heat and let the decoction steep for an additional 30 minutes.

71. Strain the decoction to remove the white willow bark pieces.

72. Optional: Add honey or lemon to taste for additional flavor.

73. Consume 1 cup of the decoction up to 3 times daily for pain relief.

Portions: Makes approximately 4 cups (950 ml), serving 4.

Beneficial Effects:

Provides natural pain relief and reduces inflammation due to the salicin content, which the body converts into salicylic acid, similar to aspirin.

Can help alleviate headaches, menstrual cramps, arthritis, and other types of pain.

Root Cause of Illness: Targets pain and inflammation by inhibiting the production of pain-inducing chemicals in the body.

Tips for Allergens:

White willow bark should be used with caution by those who are allergic to aspirin.

Individuals with a sensitivity to salicylates should consult with a healthcare provider before using white willow bark.

Honey and lemon are optional and can be omitted for those with allergies or sensitivities to these ingredients.

Activated Charcoal Cleanse Drink

Ingredients:

- 1 tablespoon activated charcoal powder (from coconut shells)
- 2 cups filtered water
- Juice of 1 lemon
- 1 tablespoon organic honey (optional, for sweetness)

Instructions:

74. In a blender, combine the activated charcoal powder with the filtered water.

75. Add the lemon juice to the mixture. If a sweeter taste is desired, include the tablespoon of honey.

76. Blend on high until all ingredients are thoroughly mixed.

77. Serve the cleanse drink immediately, or store in the refrigerator for up to 24 hours for best taste.

Portions: Makes 2 servings

Beneficial Effects:

Activated charcoal acts as a powerful detoxifier, binding to toxins and chemicals in the gut and aiding in their removal from the body.

Lemon juice adds vitamin C, supporting the immune system and enhancing the detoxifying effects of the drink.

Honey provides natural sweetness and has antimicrobial properties, further supporting the cleansing process.

Root Cause of Illness: Targets toxins and impurities in the body that can contribute to digestive issues, fatigue, and overall sluggishness by providing a natural and effective means to cleanse the digestive system.

Tips for Allergens:

Ensure the activated charcoal is food-grade and free from any additives or contaminants.

For those with allergies to citrus or honey, these ingredients can be omitted without significantly altering the detoxifying benefits of the drink.

Made in United States
Troutdale, OR
07/14/2024

21093350R10076